Volume Replacement

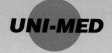

Boldt, Joachim:
Volume Replacement/Joachim Boldt.-
1. Auflage - Bremen: UNI-MED, 2004
(UNI-MED SCIENCE)
ISBN 3-89599-721-8

MEDICINE - STATE OF THE ART

UNI-MED Verlag AG, one of the leading medical publishing companies in Germany, presents its highly successful series of scientific textbooks, covering all medical subjects. The authors are specialists in their fields and present the topics precisely, comprehensively, and with the facility of quick reference in mind. The books will be most useful for all doctors who wish to keep up to date with the latest developments in medicine.

We greatly appreciate and acknowledge the collaboration of: Dr. Shreelata Datta.

Preface and acknowledgements

In the critically ill, various pathophysiological changes in systemic hemodynamics, organ blood flow, and immune function can be observed. Adequate management of the underlying insult is a prerequisite in this situation - supportive therapies including sufficient volume therapy appear to be also of importance. Recommendations on the best volume replacement regimen remain elusive. A flood of information on this topic swamps over us every year. However, we often remain "still confused, but on a much higher level" (W. Churchill). In this book, recommended experts from various disciplines cover the different aspects of "volume replacement" and "fluid substitution" and guide us through the pros and cons of the different strategies to manage our patients. Fundamental baselines, pathophysiological considerations, and recommendations for specific diseases are presented. This book is not a "cook book" for volume replacement or fluid substitution; it sums up the recent knowledge of this problem. It shows "News from the Past" as well as future aspects of volume and fluid replacement regimes. Everbody caring for the critically ill will profit from the different chapters at different levels - nurses, students, residents, consultants, and even experts on volume therapy. We should remember the origin of modern medicine: "As to diseases make a habit of two things - to help, or at least, to do no harm" (Hippocrates: Epidemic Book I, Chapter 11c. 460-377 BC)

Ludwigshafen, June 2004   *Joachim Boldt*

Authors

Prof. Dr. Joachim Boldt
Department of Anesthesiology and Intensive Care Medicine
Klinikum der Stadt Ludwigshafen
Bremserstr. 79
D-67063 Ludwigshafen
Germany
Chapter 4.3., 4.5.

Prof. Hengo Haljamäe MD, PhD
Department of Anaesthesiology and Intensive Care
The Sahlgrenska Academy at Göteborg University
Sahlgrenska University Hospital
SE-413 45 Göteborg
Sweden
Chapter 3.1.

Dr. Dirk Himpe, M.D.
Algemeen Ziekenhuis Middelheim
Campus Middelheim
Department of Anaesthesia and Intensive Care
Lindendreef 1
B-2020 Antwerp
Belgium
Chapter 4.7.

Priv.-Doz. Dr. Franz-Josef Kretz
Klinik für Anästhesiologie
und operative Intenivmedizin
Olgaspital
Bismarckstr. 8
70176 Stuttgart
Germany
Chapter 4.1.

Björn Lisander, M.D., Ph.D.
Jan Zdolsek, M.D., Ph.D.
Department of Anesthesiology
University Hospital
S-581 85 Linköping
Sweden
Chapter 4.4.

Prof. Monti Mythen
Portex Unit
6th Floor, Cardiac Wing
Institute of Child Health
30 Guliford Street
London WC1N 1EH
UK

Chapter 4.2.

Dr. Jonathan Peter Nicholson, MBBS, FRCA
Specialist Registrar in Anaesthesia
The Ipswich Hospital, Suffolk
2 Church Green
Bury St Edmunds
Suffolk, IP31 2LL
UK

Chapter 3.2.

Miss Rachel Mary Sansbury, MB BChir, MA, MRCS
Research Fellow
Department of Plastic and Reconstructive Surgery
Norfolk and Norwich University Hospital NHS Trust
Colney Lane
Norwich
NR4 7UY
UK

Chapter 3.2.

Dr. Robert Self
Centre for Anaesthesia
Room 103, The Cross Piece
University College London Hospitals
Mortimer Street
London W1T 3AA
UK

Chapter 4.2.

Univ.-Prof. Dr. Heinz Steltzer
Dept. of Anesthesia & General Intensive Care
University Hospital of Vienna
Waehringer Guertel 18-20
A-1090 Vienna
Austria

Chapter 1.

Dr. Stefan Suttner
Department of Anesthesiology and Intensive Care Medicine
Klinikum Ludwigshafen
Bremserstr. 79
D-67063 Ludwigshafen
Germany
Chapter 3.3.

Nadia Dettori, MD
Roman Kocian, MD
Donat R. Spahn, MD, FRCA
Department of Anesthesiology
University Hospital Lausanne (CHUV)
CH-1011 Lausanne
Switzerland
Chapter 3.4.

Prof. Philippe Van der Linden, MD, PhD
Department of Cardiac Anaesthesia, BT4
CHU Charleroi
Bvd Paul Janson, 92
B-6000 Charleroi
Belgium
Chapter 2.

Dr. Kristin Engelhard
Univ.-Prof. Dr. Christian Werner
Klinik für Anaesthesiologie of the Technischen Universität München
Klinikum rechts der Isar
Ismaninger Str. 22
81675 München
Germany
Chapter 4.6.

Contents

Pathophysiology of volume deficits

1. Pathophysiology of volume deficits

1.1. Introduction

Circulatory shock caused by hypovolemia is the most frequent type of clinical shock and is characterized by a reduced circulatory volume. This reduction is mainly caused by the loss of volume (blood, plasma, extravascular fluid) and supported by an interaction between mediator systems and hormones stimulated by trauma and/or tissue injury. Cardiac output is derived from heart rate, afterload, preload and contractility. Any form of inadequate cardiac output associated with inadequate blood flow to tissues can be defined as shock. Normally, shock is accompanied by low blood pressure and reduced venous return. Blood flow to individual tissues is determined by blood pressure and regional resistance of the vessels. Blood pressure is important for the maintenance of perfusion since it takes blood through the different regions of the body. By simplifying Poiseuille's law, arterial pressure is the product of cardiac output and systemic vascular resistance. Causes of low systemic vascular resistance are sepsis, arteriovenous shunts and several drugs. Decrease in cardiac output may be caused by decreased cardiac function (myopathy, infarction), sepsis or drugs. A reduced venous return is related to decreased mean systemic filling pressure and intravascular volume. The volume that describes the mean systemic pressure in addition to the compliance of the peripheral circuit is named "stressed volume" and the volume that does not do so is called "unstressed volume". As a consequence, during hemorrhage, the loss of stressed volume will result in a decrease of mean systemic pressure and this produces a decrease of venous return in any right arterial pressure. An increase in peripheral vascular resistance will restore blood pressure but will not change bad perfusion of peripheral tissues. Consequently, cardiac output can only be changed by altering the determinants of venous return (i.e. stressed volume, vascular compliance and resistance). Venous return can be increased by either increasing precapillary resistance or decreasing postcapillary resistance that will result in a shift of fluid from the interstitial space to the intravascular characterized by a decrease in hematocrit and that necessary for long term adjustments after hemorrhage. Venous return can also be changed by decreasing venous compliance or a decrease in unstressed volume, leading to a leftward shift in the pressure volume curve (1).

> The most frequent clinical relevant etiologies of hypovolemia are trauma, dehydration (gastrointestinal losses), and sepsis. Early resuscitation of patients with severe hypovolemia or hypovolemic shock should be made in time since any delay results in organ dysfunction (cardiac, renal, liver) and sometimes in irreversible states of shock. Therefore in clinical practice, resuscitation of these patients goes in time with evaluation of the underlying etiology.

1.2. Consequences of hypovolemia

Cardiac function during hypovolemia is related to the degree of volume loss and to the influence of mediators according to the underlying causes. The most common cause of heart failure in shock is a distinct reduction of the venous return due to hypovolemia. If the hypovolemia is severe or persists over a longer period of time, compensatory changes in autonomic function of the heart (contractility, heart rate) may be insufficient and progressive circulatory failure will be the result. After a mild loss of blood volume (10 %) a decrease in filling pressures and the enddiastolic area results in a minor decrease in preload thereby causing lower stroke volume and cardiac output. The concomitant fall in arterial pressure and reduction in baroreceptor activity promotes increasing myocardial contractility and heart rate. Consequently, stroke volume increases at lower cardiac filling pressures accompanied by elevated oxygen demand of the myocardium and reduction in coronary resistance. Moderate hypovolemia (lack of around 25 % of the circulating blood volume) induces further increases in contractility and heart rate together with systemic vasoconstriction but leads to a reduction in cardiac output and to elevations of myocardial oxygen consumption. Ischemic damage and the release of proinflammatory mediators (like the myocardial depressant factor) might play a role during these conditions. Further blood loss or hypovolemia causes in most cases a linear decline in arterial blood pressure and fall in cardiac output. Myocardial compensatory mechanisms are inadequate and the renin-angiotensin-system is highly activated in order to preserve water and salt. Finally, myocardial ischemia, arrhythmias and pump failure are evident (2).

Acute hypovolemia is normally compensated by complex endocrine responses. After activation of the renin-angiotensin-aldosteron systems the release of vasopressin - a potent vasoconstrictor - occurs and produces increasing reabsorption of water from the renal system and as a second effect, induces vasoconstriction in the splanchnic system. In addition, lipolysis and gluconeogenesis result in a hyperglycemia and insulin resistance which by themselves produce a hyperosmolarity of the blood and fluid shifts from intracellular to the intravascular space. The renin-angiotensin system stimulated by beta-adrenergic receptors or due to decreased preload stimulated by the renal arterioles leads to the production of renin and circulating angiotensins I and II. The predominant target of the latter is the production of vasoconstriction (increased afterload, reduced compliance of the heart), and, after aldosterone secretion, angiotensin II induces salt and water retention with subsequent increase in intravascular volume and preload (3).

Besides activation of various inflammatory mediators and vasoactive substances, the endothelium plays a central role by influencing the vascular tone. The microcirculatory interaction of nitric oxide, endothelins, prostaglandins and angiotensin II is involved in the regulation of microcirculatory blood flow. Therefore, hypovolemia and hypovolemic shock are triggered off by certain insults (i.e. pain, infection or local trauma) and are accompanied by both neural and humoral stimuli and result in typical clinical symptoms such as acidosis, hypotension and metabolic disorders.

Neurohormonal effects in response to hypovolemia associated with increasing central vasoconstriction should support adequate cardiac preload and circulating blood volume for oxygenation of the heart and brain. As a consequence, inadequate early treatment of shock and hypoperfusion (i.e. application of catecholamine instead of ade-

quate volume loading) may support the vicious circle and should definitely be avoided.

> Treatment strategies of hyovolemia should be more or less standardized. Firstly adequate venous access and early institution of blood volume monitoring and secondly fluid resuscitation using crystalloid/colloid solutions are recommended.

1.3. Hypovolemia in the polytrauma patient

In patients with polytrauma the primary goal of the circulatory treatment should be the prevention of any progression into a hypodynamic state of shock. Therefore, the immediate use of fluid and catecholamine support is of central importance. If we cannot reach a hyperdynamic state of circulation, regional perfusion deficits caused by inadequate oxygen extraction can facilitate the development of organ dysfunction. The reduction of blood volume of less than 10 % will be compensated without distinct changes of cardiac output. Otherwise decreasing preload, cardiac output and arterial pressure are typical signs of reduced oxygen delivery. In order to ensure the adequacy of circulatory blood volume, we need definite guidelines. Previous guidelines have proposed to use changes in central venous pressure (CVP) or pulmonary capillary wedge pressure (PCWP) to predict the response to fluid application (incremental increases of CVP of more than 5 mmHg, PCWP between 12 and 16 mmHg or enddiastolic volume of more than 110 mL). It is essential that volume replacement is given rapidly so that losses into the interstitial space are low. This is only possible when large central venous or peripheral venous accesses are used. A more rapidly infused volume remains longer in the vascular space and increases stressed volume. Volume expansion is only effective as long as the right heart is responsive to changes in right ventricular enddiastolic volume (RVEDV) which has not reached the flat part of the cardiac function curve. If this is the case, a further increase in (stressed) blood volume will result in unchanged cardiac output. The pressure for reaching this plateau depends on various clinical conditions. It may be high in patients with pulmonary hypertension and decreased compliance of the right heart, moderately high during left ventricular dilatation and interventricular interdependence, and low in normal subjects. Therefore using monitoring of end-diastolic volume seems to be the best way of observing the results of fluid challenges. Normally, in the first days after trauma, patients may need a positive fluid balance for the replacement of losses into the third space or interstitium until the backshift of fluid starts some days after the trauma. After injury, the neuroendocrine response is characterized by vasoconstriction, resulting in reduced capacity of the cardiocirculatory system followed by an increase in venous return to the heart. Blood flow to the brain and the heart is maintained as long as possible by arteriolar vasoconstriction and increased peripheral total vascular resistance. This global vasoconstriction is not uniform since a marked redistribution of regional blood flow can occur. On the one hand, the maintenance of regional perfusion in heart and brain will be supported by metabolic vasoregulation and increasing activities of the vasomotor center in the medulla. On the other hand, triggered by acute hypovolemia, regional blood flow to splanchnic circulation, skeletal muscle, skin and other nonessential tissues is reduced and sometimes associated with a decreased renal blood flow. As a result, acute renal dysfunction with oliguria or anuria will be a useful parameter for monitoring of hypovolemia. In general, the splanchnic region is very sensitive to hypovolemia and hypotension and may lead to a progression of the impairment of the gut barrier function allowing further translocation and initiation of sepsis (4).

1.4. Hypovolemia and sepsis

Hypovolemia during sepsis and septic shock is characterized by low peripheral resistance and higher cardiac output with decreased blood pressure but increased venous return. This is may be caused by an increase in the unstressed volume related to the decreasing total vascular volume. The increase of cardiac output in order to augment oxygen delivery is one of the important goals in septic patients. Stressed volume, however, is a major determinant of venous return and should be replaced in time by using fluids. Usually, patients will need several liters of fluid to increase filling pressures and cardiac output. The capillary leak causes rapid fluid losses into the interstitial space. As a consequence, the increase of mean systemic pressure by means of norepinephrine can be performed by decreasing unstressed volume and increasing stressed volume. This might be associated with increasing renal blood flow and urinary output.

1.5. The dehydrated patient

During several phases of dehydration, the normal body is able to compensate the resulting hypovolemia by redistributing fluid from "peripheral" organs (skin, muscles, splanchnic circulation and renal) to "central" organs like brain or heart. During hypovolemia, the loss of circulatory blood volume is associated with a decrease in cardiac output and systolic arterial pressure. In order to prevent the progress to a fatal scenario of inadequate tissue perfusion, the cardiovascular system is able to control the effectiveness of blood flow. This includes the hormonal response to volume depletion, the control of cardiac performance and contractility and some approaches of organ specific regulations of regional blood flow. The endothelial dysfunction may play an important role in septic patients and is characterized by peripheral vascular paralysis, impaired regulation of blood flow, endothelial injury with increased endothelial permeability, interstitial edema and loss of plasma proteins. In this group of patients, hypoperfusion per se is a distinct activator of systemic inflammatory response and together with endotoxins and other shock mediators function as a contributor to the multiple organ dysfunction. This complex pathophysiological process is a mirror of inadequate oxygenation due to low perfusion of the tissues. Adequate volume replacement appears essential for the improvement of the microcirculatory nutritive blood flow and consequently the reduction or avoidance of damaging inflammatory cascades.

1.6. Hypovolemia in burns

Destruction of the skin after burns injury is followed by a superoxide-mediated destruction of the skin barrier and production of necrotic tissue. This leads to the initiation of an inflammatory response including the activation of neutrophils, endothelial cells and mediators (i.e. histamine, prostaglandins, cytokines, endothelin). A characteristic sign of the inflammatory response is the development of edema, followed by vasodilatation. As a consequence, severe hypovolemia and hypotension will occur if fluid application is not rapidly established. Further abnormalities are high levels of albumin in the capillary system and increased absorption of the interstitial area leading to severe hypovolemia. As clinical manifestations, vasoconstriction, hypoalbuminemia, hyponatremia and cardiac dysfunction may occur. Despite adequate substitution with crystalloids, buffer solutions and albumin, a hyperkinetic shock may occur with metabolic acidosis, tachycardia and some decrease in systemic vascular resistance. Acute burn injury is followed by immediate release of proinflammatory cytokines, hypermetabolism and distinct fluid shifts. The fluid resuscitation should consider that on the one hand, a release of thromboxane with pulmonary hypertension may cause a right and left ventricular failure whether or not a "myocardial depressant" factor may play a supporting role. On the other hand, hypermetabolism stimulated by the first hit of burning trauma is responsible for increasing peripheral oxygen demand and subsequent oxygen delivery. Prevention or early treatment of deleterious effects of burn injury on the cardiovascular system should be the superior goal in this setting. The extent of injury and the size of the patient are major determinants of the resuscitation volume to produce adequate tissue perfusion. Although burn resuscitation formulas are used to provide an estimation of requirement, further consideration is important. While one group of authors points towards the importance of clinical parameter for guiding resuscitation (blood pressure, heart rate, urine output) others are stressing the clinical importance of accurate measurements using invasive monitoring and derived parameters.

1.7. Monitoring of hypovolemia

Although patients with hypovolemia due to surgery or trauma rapidly reveal oxygen debts signaled by increased base deficits and lactate levels, studies of resuscitation with fluid and higher doses of catecholamines to achieve supranormal values for oxygen transport are unable to show a better survival rate. On the other hand, traditional endpoints of resuscitation, such as heart rate, blood pressure, central venous pressure, and urinary output failed to differentiate between surviving and nonsurviving patients.

For the management of hypovolemic patients independent of the etiology not only is the assessment of preload important, it is also the responsiveness of patients to a volume application and/or other cardiovascular interventions. Measurements of arterial and central venous pressures are the first level for estimation of preload, since right arterial and right ventricular enddiastolic pressure are partly reflected by this parameter. However, the responsiveness to fluid will not be predicted. Over the last 30 years, the pulmonary capillary wedge pressure (PCWP) measured by the Swan Ganz catheter has been the "gold standard" for invasive monitoring of preload. The assumption of equality of left arterial pressure and pulmonary capillary wedge pressure reflects the fact that the left ventricular preload has been the basis of interpretation. Further developments and modifications allowed monitoring of right ventricular ejection fraction (RVEF) and enddiastolic volume (RVEDV), and as the most accurate tool, more or less continuous measurements of cardiac output together with mixed venous saturation. However, insufficient knowledge of physicians paired with the fact that the perioperative use has no benefit for patients' outcome (5) was the basis for decreasing clinical applications of pulmonary artery catheters.

By using another concept concentrating on pulse contour analysis in addition to a central venous and a (femoral) arterial access, all relevant hemodynamic parameters can be obtained. Using a PiCCO device, calculation of beat-by-beat cardiac output from arterial waveform and intrathoracic blood volume (ITBV) which summarizes blood volumes from left and right heart plus pulmonary blood, is possible. This may represent a more reliable calculation of preload. Furthermore, the cardiac function index (contractile function), extravascular lung water (EVLW, pulmonary edema) and stroke volume variation (SVV, volume responsiveness during controlled ventilation) are additional parameters for guiding fluid therapy. The assessment of responsiveness to a fluid challenge seems to be a particularly reliable clinical tool. In contrast to pressure and area analysis, systolic pressure variations were considered as good indicators for changes in stroke volume and therefore as a good predictor for the responsiveness to fluid therapy (6). Recent studies have shown that left ventricular response to fluid load was related to the quantification of systolic pressure variations and that by means of these variables, occult hypovolemia may be detectable early (7). Despite these encouraging results, new monitoring devices for guiding fluid replacement or resuscitation have to be evaluated and compared with "gold standard" monitoring techniques.

> Invasive monitoring may be helpful to avoid inadequate volume replacement and suboptimal resuscitation.

For monitoring of circulating blood volume, various techniques are clinically applicable. Besides the right ventricular catheter with all advantages and side effects, a new generation of semi-invasive tools is now available. According to recent literature, volume application in sepsis-related hypovolemia can be guided either with pulmonary artery catheter (PAC) - derived enddiastolic volumes together with changes in mixed venous saturation or venous saturation alone, or by using the PICCO-system and derived calculations such as global end-diastolic volume, intrathoracic blood volume and extravascular lung water (8). In addition to goals guided by these monitoring-tools, there are proposed goals for resuscitation in trauma patients according to the recommendation of big centers with experience in resuscitation of this subgroup of patients. These goals include systolic blood pressure of 80 mmHg or more, heart rate less than 120 beats/min, peripheral oxygen saturation of more than 96 %, urine output of more than 0.5 mL/kg/h, hemoglobin >9 g/dl, lactate levels < 1,6 mmol/l, base deficit of more than -5 with the ability of patients to follow simple commands accurately (9).

Since the splanchnic region may be essentially involved in the hypovolemic stages of shock assessments of changes in regional CO_2 by means of tonometric devices could give us additional information about the effectiveness of fluid resuscitation (10).

> In summary, the body has a variety of possibilities to counteract hypovolemic insults, but the early detection of hypovolemia appears essential for the management of hypovolemic patients or patients with shock. Although fluid challenge and replacement is a first choice therapy, not all patients will be responders to fluid alone, others would benefit from additional inotropic support or use of vasopressors. The underlying cause of hypovolemia or shock may play an essential role for the planning of the subsequent management. In this context, use of adequate monitoring for assessing the severity of hypovolemia and the responsiveness to volume load appears important.

1.8. References

1. Guyton AC. Textbook of Medical Physiology. Philadelphia: WB Saunders, 1991

2. Schlag G, Redl H (eds). Pathophysiology of Shock, Sepsis, and Organ failure. Berlin: Springer Verlag 1993

3. Cerra FB (ed). Manual of Critical Care. St Louis: CV Mosby 1987

4. Pinsky MR, Dhainaut JF (eds). Pathophysiologic Foundations of Critical Care. Baltimore: Williams & Willkins 1993

5. Sandham JD, Hull RD, Brant RF et al. A randomized controlled trial of the use of pulmonary artery catheters in high risk surgical patients. New Engl J Med 2003; 348:5-14

6. Rodig G, Prasser C, Keyl C et al. Continuous cardiac output measurement pulse contour analysis vs thermodilution technique in cardiac surgical patients. Br J Anaesth 1999; 4: 525-530

7. Tavernier B, Makothine O, Lebuffe G et al. Systolic pressure variation as a guide to fluid therapy in patients with sepsis- induced hypotension. Anesthesiology 1998; 89:1313-1321

8. Michard F, Teboul JL. Predicting fluid responsiveness in ICU Patients- a critical analysis of the evidence. Chest 2002; 121:2000-2008

9. McCunn M, Dutton R. Endpoints of resuscitation: how much is enough? Curr Opin Anaesthesiol 2000; 13:147-153

10. Ivatury RR, Simon RJ, Havriliak D, Garcia D, Greenbarg J, Stahl WM. Gastric mucosal pH and oxygen delivery and oxygen consumption indices in the assessement of adequacy of resuscitation after trauma: a prospective, randomized study. J Trauma 1995; 39:128-136

Blood and blood derivatives

2. Blood and blood derivatives

Circulating blood volume is an important, but often unmeasured variable in intensive care unit (ICU) patients and in patients undergoing major surgery (1). Alterations in vascular volume, which are common in the surgical and the ICU patient, can influence hemoglobin (Hb) concentrations and may affect their interpretation; a patient with an apparently normal hemoglobin level but who is dehydrated may, in fact, be more compromised than a patient with a low hemoglobin level who is hemodiluted but has adequate circulating blood volume.

Severe volume depletion leads to clearly recognizable clinical shock that requires urgent intervention. Smaller volume depletion can be less recognizable since sympathetic-mediated vasoconstriction allows redistribution of blood flow to vital organs. Despite the maintenance of arterial blood pressure, reduced blood flow to several organs such as the kidney and gastrointestinal tract may render them ischemic. Untreated hypovolemia also leads to exaggerated inflammatory and immune responses that can result in the development of a systemic inflammatory response syndrome. This syndrome shares many clinical features of bacterial sepsis (2). Therefore, in high-risk patients, even relatively small volume depletion can have serious physiological consequences. Several studies showed that preoperative plasma volume expansion aimed at optimising circulating blood volume could help to prevent the development of regional hypoxia (3,4).

Blood and blood derivatives occupy a special place in the context of volume replacement strategies. Although not actually administered to increase circulating blood volume, they can contribute to it. Blood derivates such as fresh frozen plasma (FFP) and platelet concentrates are specifically administered to treat or to prevent bleeding disorders. They have absolutely no indication for volume replacement in any circumstances. The administration of FFP in sufficient amounts to restore adequate clotting factors levels (10-15 mL/kg) could, however, represent a significant volume of fluid that has to be taken into account when assessing a patient's fluid balance. The aims of allogeneic blood transfusion in ICU patients are to reduce the

risks associated with anemia and/or to increase oxygen delivery (DO_2) in an attempt to improve survival in these critically ill patients. In an evaluation of transfusion practice in tertiary-level intensive care units, Hébert et al. (5) reported that the most frequent reasons for administering red blood cells were bleeding and the need to augment oxygen delivery. Clearly, the decision to transfuse a given patient requires taking into account not only the risks related to anemia but also the risk-benefit ratios of erythrocyte transfusion. As hemodynamic optimisation in high-risk patients might improve outcome, this chapter will focus on the use of red blood cell (RBC) transfusion within the context of oxygen delivery optimisation.

2.1. Oxygen delivery in the high-risk patient

The delivery of oxygen from the environment to the cell entails a sequence of convective and diffusive stages in which oxygen is transported through the lungs, carried in the blood, and unloaded in the tissues. The regulation of this delivery, through the control of ventilation, and the regulation and distribution of cardiac output, normally allows oxygen consumption (VO_2) to proceed at a rate set by tissue oxygen demand in response to its metabolic activity (6). The complex mechanisms that regulate the matching of tissue oxygen delivery to tissue oxygen demand are frequently altered in the critically ill, resulting in the development of tissue hypoxia. Tissue hypoxia, caused by an imbalance between oxygen demand and oxygen uptake of the peripheral tissues, is considered an important contributing factor to the morbidity and mortality observed in critically ill patients. Confirming the findings published by Clowes and Del Guercio in 1960 (7), many studies have repeatedly reported that survivors of major operations had consistently higher cardiac output and oxygen delivery than those patients who subsequently died (8). Based on these observations, one approach to prevent or to correct tissue hypoxia in critically ill patients has been to increase global oxygen delivery to levels associated with survival from critical illness.

A number of randomised clinical trials (RCTs) have tested the hypothesis that optimisation of oxygen delivery is associated with decreased mortality and morbidity in critically ill patients. The results of these trials are conflicting and have generated considerable controversy. RCTs can be classified into two groups: those that adopted a prophylactic approach, i.e., early adoption of interventions in an attempt to prevent tissue hypoxia and those that adopted a concurrent approach, i.e., later adoption of interventions in an attempt to correct tissue hypoxia (9). Interestingly, most studies that described decreased mortality with optimisation of DO_2 used a prophylactic approach while those using the concurrent approach reported variable results. These observations are consistent with the hypothesis that optimisation of DO_2 may decrease mortality by preventing the development of tissue hypoxia, but is less effective in lowering mortality when used to reverse tissue hypoxia. There is indeed growing evidence that optimisation of oxygen delivery in high-risk patients to prevent the development of tissue hypoxia leads to improved outcome (10-16). There is, however, limited consensus on which patients are most likely to benefit from increased global oxygen delivery. It also remains to be elucidated whether the potential benefits related to preoperative oxygen delivery optimisation can be achieved by increased intravenous fluid therapy alone or whether it is necessary for some patients to receive supplemental inotropic/vasodilator agents (17). Of note, all published RCTs evaluating the effects of oxygen delivery optimisation maintained hemoglobin concentrations above 10 g/dL. Hence, inferences regarding the potential therapeutic effect of RBC transfusion in this context were not possible.

2.2. Efficacy of red blood cell transfusion

Eighteen clinical studies for a total of 359 patients attempted to determine the effect of RBC transfusion on the VO_2 DO_2 relationship (18-35). All measured VO_2 and DO_2 before and after the transfusion of a specified number of allogeneic RBC units. The results of these trials, shown in Table 2.1, are inconsistent.

Although Hb concentration increased significantly in all the studies, DO_2 did not increase in four of them. Despite the administration of 1 to 3 RBC units, cardiac filling pressures did not increase, and

cardiac output did not change or even decrease. Indeed, acute hemoconcentration will be associated with an exponential increase in blood viscosity at all shear rates, particularly at the lowest ones prevalent in the postcapillary venules. This phenomenon will result in a decrease in venous return at the systemic level (36) as well as a reduction in bulk flow (37). At the microcirculatory level, it translates into a reduction of mean red blood cell velocity and an increased number of capillaries containing stationary RBCs (38). Therefore, in the studies reporting an increase in DO_2 with blood transfusion, this elevation was essentially related to a rise in arterial blood oxygen content.

In the 14 studies that showed an increase in systemic DO_2, only five reported an increase in systemic VO_2 (18,21,29,30,33). Blood lactate levels were not predictive of VO_2 changes given that only two of the eight studies (18,19,22,23,25,27,30,33) evaluating patients with increased lactate concentration noted an increase in VO_2 (18,30). In addition, the studies that demonstrated an increase in VO_2 should be interpreted with caution since in all of them VO_2 was calculated using the Fick equation. Calculating both VO_2 and DO_2 from the same values of cardiac output, arterial saturation and hemoglobin concentration may indeed introduce a problem of mathematical coupling of the data. This phenomenon is more likely to occur when DO_2 variations associated with therapeutic interventions are of small amplitude (39). The three studies that directly measured VO_2 (25,27,31) did not report an increase in VO_2 associated with blood transfusion, although two of them did show a significant increase in calculated VO_2 (25,31).

From a physiological standpoint, the lack of a VO_2 change in the presence of a significant increase in DO_2 could be attributed either to the absence of an oxygen deficit or to the inability of RBC transfusion to correct a tissue oxygenation debt. The evaluation of blood transfusion effects on VO_2 requires, therefore, situations in which VO_2 DO_2 dependency can be identified. Two recent experimental studies specifically address this issue. In rats subjected to supply-dependency conditions by acute isovolemic anemia, Fitzgerald et al. (40) and Sielenkämper et al. (41) demonstrated that the transfusion of rat blood stored for 28 days increases hemoglobin concentration, but fails to correct tissue hypoxia when compared with fresh rat blood (sto-

	Patients	Death (%)	Transfusion Hb (g/dL)	VO₂ Measure	Lactate	DO₂	VO₂
Sepsis & septic shock							
Gilbert et al., 1986 (18)	17 (65 ± 17 y)	75	NA 8.7 - 11.3	Indirect	Normal Increased	⇑ ⇑	⇔ ⇑
Conrad et al., 1990 (19)	19 (44 ± 5 y)	NA	591 ± 55 mL 8.3 - 10.7	Indirect	Increased	⇑	⇔
Mink et al., 1990 (20)	8 (2 mo - 6 y)	37	8 -10 mL/kg 10.2 - 13.2	Indirect	NA	⇑	⇔
Lucking et al., 1990 (21)	7 (4 mo - 15 y)	NA	10 - 15 mL/kg 9.3 - 12.4	Indirect	NA	⇑	⇑
Dietrich et al., 1990 (22)	32 (1 - 77 y)	NA	70 - 1400 mL 8.3 - 10.5	Indirect	Increased	⇑	⇔
Steffes et al., 1991 (33)	21 (37 - 83 y)	67	1 - 2 units 9.3 - 10.7	Indirect	Normal Increased	⇑ ⇑	⇑ ⇔
Silverman et al., 1992 (23)	21 (21 - 88 y)	38	2 units 8.5 - 10.7	Indirect	Increased	⇑	⇔
Lorente et al., 1993 (24)	16	62.5	800 mL 9.6 - 11.6	Indirect	NA	⇑	⇔
Marik et al., 1993 (25)	23 (20 - 79 y)	71	3 units 9.0 -11.9	Direct	NA	⇑	⇔
Gramm et al., 1996 (26)	19 (46 ± 3 y)	0	2 units 8.4 - 10.1	Indirect	Normal Increased	⇔	⇔
Fernandes et al., 2001 (27)	10 (18 - 80 y)	70	1 unit 9.4 - 10.1	Direct	Normal	⇔	⇔
Acute respiratory failure							
Kahn et al., 1986 (28)	15	NA	7 mL/kg 10.9 - 12.5	Indirect	NA	⇔	⇔
Ronco et al., 1990 (29)	5 (20 - 47 y)	100	2 units 10.9 - 13	Indirect	NA	⇑	⇑
Fenwick et al., 1990 (30)	24 (38 - 66 y)	55	2 units 9.8 - 12.0	Indirect	Normal Increased	⇑ ⇑	⇔ ⇑
Ronco et al., 1991 (31)	17 (20 - 70 y)	71	2 units	Direct	NA	⇑	⇔
Postoperative & post-trauma							
Shah et al., 1982 (32)	8 (28 – 76 y)	NA	2 units 9.2 - 11.1	Indirect	NA	⇔	⇔
Babineau et al., 1992 (34)	30 (33 – 86 y)	NA	1 unit 9.4 - 10.4	Indirect	NA	⇑	⇔
Casutt et al., 1999 (35)	67 (32 - 81 y)	NA	368 ± 10 mL 8.1 - 9.0	Indirect	NA	⇑	⇔

Table 2.1: Effects of RBC transfusion on global O₂ balance, NA : not announced.

red < 3 days). The inability of old transfused red blood cells to acutely augment systemic VO_2 from a supply-dependent position can be explained by the structural and functional changes in the RBC product occurring with storage. RBC 2,3 diphosphoglycerate (2,3 DPG) concentration decreases to near zero after two weeks of storage, and then regenerates after transfusion at a variable rate (from one to several days) (17). This reduction in intracellular 2,3 DPG results in a left shift in the oxyhaemoglobin dissociation curve, reducing the ability of transfused RBCs to offload oxygen to the tissues. During storage, there is also a progressive decrease in adenosine triphosphate (ATP), which is accompanied by a change in RBC shape from discoid to spherocytic, a loss of membrane lipid, and a decrease in cellular deformability (42). Reduced RBC deformability will also diminish tissue oxygen availability by impeding access to the capillary network and by increasing blood viscosity (36,43). In conjunction with significant systemic microcirculatory dysfunction observed in many critical illnesses (44,45), the decrease in RBC deformability may dramatically affect tissue oxygen delivery in these high-risk patients.

Systemic VO_2 is the algebraic sum of oxygen consumption in individual organs. Unchanged whole body VO_2 measurements may obscure the presence of significant VO_2 changes in individual organs. Marik *et al.* (25) measured gastric intramucosal pH (pHi), an indicator of gut mucosal oxygenation, in septic patients to determine whether significant changes could be demonstrated at the organ level while not simultaneously reflected by whole body VO_2 measurements. They reported a decrease in the pHi of patients transfused with RBCs that had been stored for more than 15 days, confirming previous observations that gut oxygen availability may decrease paradoxically following blood transfusion (23). The authors hypothesized that the transfusion of old, poorly deformable RBCs could lead to microcapillary sludging and obstruction, thereby reducing nutritive gut oxygen delivery in patients presenting with sepsis-related microcirculatory alterations (45). These findings may have important clinical implications given the increasing attention focused on the role of the gut in both the initiation and propagation of the patient's septic response. The deleterious effects of "old" RBC transfusion on gut oxygen delivery could also be related to the volume of blood transfused. For example, Fernandes *et al.* (27) did not observe a worsening of pHi after the transfusion of only one RBC unit in septic patients whereas Marik *et al.* (25) did after the transfusion of 3 units.

Even if "fresh" RBC transfusion proved to be effective in restoring VO_2 in supply-dependent conditions, its efficacy would have to be compared with other standard forms of treatment aimed at augmenting DO_2, such as increasing blood flow. From a physiological point of view, increased blood flow could theoretically augment the perfused capillary area by increases in filling pressure or microvascular vasodilation, thus resulting in increased oxygen uptake. The effects of blood transfusion may be less predictable as the rise in hematocrit will increase blood viscosity, which, in turn, may alter regional microvascular blood flow (36). This issue was addressed in a canine model of cardiopulmonary bypass (46). Using a randomised two-period crossover design, this study compared the efficacy of "fresh" (stored < 3 days) RBC transfusion and increased blood flow to restore tissue oxygenation in oxygen supply-dependent conditions. Both techniques produced a similar increase in DO_2 and were equally effective in restoring tissue oxygenation. These results are in contrast with those reported by Lorente *et al.* (24). In patients with severe sepsis, only the increase in blood flow produced by dobutamine resulted in an increase in VO_2. However, in this study, the DO_2 increase obtained with dobutamine was higher than the one realized with blood transfusion. In addition, the increase in VO_2 observed with dobutamine may be attributable to its direct calorigenic effects. Finally, the age of the RBCs transfused was not specified.

2.3. Conclusion

Although RBC transfusion is usually administered to increase whole body DO_2, this is not always the case, as the rise in oxygen-carrying capacity may be counterbalanced by a decrease in blood flow secondary to increased blood viscosity. Even in the presence of increased systemic DO_2, RBC transfusion may not result in greater oxygen availability to the cells owing to the effects of storage on RBC membrane deformability and on the affinity of hemoglobin for oxygen. These effects on tissue oxygen availability are probably even more marked in critically ill patients, who already present with si-

gnificant microcirculatory dysfunction and reduced RBC deformability associated with the inflammatory reaction. In view of the available literature,
the liberal use of RBC transfusion to maintain systemic DO_2 at high levels in critically ill patients is
no longer justified. Hébert *et al.* (47) demonstrated
that a restrictive RBC transfusion strategy (Hb between 7 and 9 g/dL) is at least as effective as, and
possibly superior to, a liberal transfusion strategy
(Hb between 10 and 12 g/dL) in volume-
resuscitated critically ill patients. The failure of old
RBC transfusion to acutely improve tissue oxygen
availability could have therapeutic implications for
the quality of blood transfused, especially when an
improvement in tissue oxygenation is desired. The
most straightforward approach would be to transfuse freshly donated blood. Such an approach, however, would result in major organizational problems for blood transfusion centers. Another approach would be to develop treatments that either
protect or restore RBC properties before transfusion. Future studies are needed to determine if the
development of such strategies will help to reduce
mortality and morbidity when the cellular oxygen
supply is threatened.

2.4. References

1. Jones JG, Wardrop AJ. Measurement of blood volume
in surgical and intensive care practice. Br J Anaesth 2000;
84: 226-35

2. Gosling P, Bascom JU, Zikria BA. Capillary leak, oedema and organ failure. Care Crit 1996; 12: 191-7

3. Mythen MG, Webb AR. Preoperative plasma volume
expansion reduces the incidence of gut mucosal hypoperfusion during cardiac surgery. Arch Surg 1995; 130:
423-9

4. Sinclair S, James S, Singer M. Intraoperative intravascular volume optimisation and length of hospital stay after repair of proximal femoral fracture: randomised controlled trial. Br Med J 1997; 315: 909-12

5. Hébert PC, Wells G, Marshall J, Martin C, Tweeddale
MG, Pagliarello G, Blajchman MA. Transfusion requirement in critical care: a pilot study. JAMA 1995; 273:
1439-44

6. Schumacker PT, Cain SM. The concept of a critical
oxygen delivery. Intensive Care Med 1987; 13: 223-9

7. Clowes GHA, Del Guercio LRM. Circulatory response
to the trauma of surgical operations. Metabolism 1960;
9: 67-81

8. Grounds RM, Rhodes A, Bennet ED. Reducing mortality and complications, 2001 Yearbook of Intensive Care
and Emergency Medicine. Edited by Vincent J-L. Berlin
Heidelberg, Springer Verlag, 2001, pp 57-67

9. Russel JA. Adding fuel to the fire - The supranormal
oxygen delivery trials controversy. Crit Care Med 1998;
26: 981-3

10. Shoemaker WC, Appel PL, Kram HB, Waxman K,
Lee T-S. Prospective trial of supranormal values of survi-
vors as therapeutic goals in high-risk surgical patients.
Chest 1988; 94: 1176-86

11. Berlauk JF, Abrams JH, Gilmour IJ, O'Connor SR,
Knighton DR, Cerra FB. Preoperative optimization of
cardiovascular hemodynamics improves outcome in peripheral vascular surgery. A prospective randomized clinical trial. Ann Surg 1991; 214: 289-99

12. Boyd O, Grounds M, Bennet ED. A randomized clinical trial of the effect of deliberate perioperative increase
of oxygen delivery on mortality in high risk surgical patients. JAMA 1993; 270: 2699-707

13. Wilson J, Woods I, Fawcett J, Whall R, Dibb W, Morris C, McManus E. Reducing the risk of major elective
surgery: randomised controlled trial of preoperative optimisation of oxygen delivery. Br Med J 1999; 318: 1099-
103

14. Lobo SMA, Salgado PF, Castillo VGT, Borim AA, Po-
lachini CA, Palchetti JC, Brienzi SLA, de Oliveira GG. Effects of maximizing oxygen delivery on morbidity and
mortality in high-risk surgical patients. Crit Care Med
2000; 28: 3396-404

15. Heyland DK, Cook DJ, King D, Kerneman P, Brun-
Buisson C. Maximizing oxygen delivery in critically ill
patients: a methodologic appraisal of the evidence. Crit
Care Med 1996; 24: 517-24

16. Rivers E, Nguyen B, Havstad S, Ressler J, Muzzin A,
Knoblich B, Peterson E, Tomlanovich M. Early goal-
directed therapy in the treatment of severe sepsis and
septic shock. N Engl J Med 2001; 345: 1368-77

17. Hébert PC. Red cell transfusion strategies in the ICU.
Vox Sang 2000; 78: 167-77

18. Gilbert EM, Haupt MT, Mandanas RY, Huaringa AJ,
Carlson RW. The effect of fluid loading, blood transfusion and catecholamine infusion on oxygen delivery and
consumption in patients with sepsis. Am Rev Respir Dis
1986; 134: 873-8

19. Conrad SA, Dietrich KA, Hebert CA, Romero MD.
Effect of red blood cell transfusion on oxygen consumption following fluid resuscitation in septic shock. Circulatory Shock 1990; 31: 419-29

20. Mink RB, Pollack MM. Effect of blood transfusion on
oxygen consumption in pediatric septic shock. Crit Care
Med 1990; 18: 1087-91

21. Lucking SE, Williams TM, Chaten FC, Metz RI, Mickell JJ. Dependence of oxygen consumption on oxygen delivery in children with hyperdynamic septic shock and low oxygen extraction. Crit Care Med 1990; 18: 1316-9

22. Dietrich KA, Conrad SA, Hebert CA: Cardiovascular and metabolic response to red blood cell transfusion in critically ill volume-resuscitated nonsurgical patients. Crit Care Med 1990; 18: 940-5

23. Silverman HJ, Tuma P. Gastric tonometry in patients with sepsis: effects of dobutamine infusion and packed red blood cell transfusions. Chest 1992; 102: 184-8

24. Lorente JA, Landin L, De Pablo R, Renes E, Rodriguez-Diaz R, Liste D. Effects of blood transfusion on oxygen transport variables in severe sepsis. Crit Care Med 1993; 21: 1312-8

25. Marik PE, Sibbald WJ. Effects of stored blood transfusion on oxygen delivery in patients with sepsis. JAMA 1993; 269: 3024-9

26. Gramm J, Smith S, Gamelli RL, Dries DJ. Effect of transfusion on oxygen transport in critically ill patients. Shock 1996; 5: 190-3

27. Fernandes Jr CF, Akamine N, De Marco FVC, De Souza JAM, Lagudis S, Knobel E. Red blood cell transfusion does not increase oxygen consumption in critically ill septic patients. Critical Care 2001; 5: 362-7

28. Kahn RC, Zaroulis C, Goetz W, Howland WS. Hemodynamic oxygen transport and 2,3-diphosphoglycerate changes after transfusion of patients with acute respiratory failure. Intensive Care Med 1986; 12: 22-5

29. Ronco JJ, Montaner JSG, Fenwick JC, Ruedy J, Russel JA. Pathologic dependence of oxygen consumption on oxygen delivery in acute respiratory failure secondary to AIDS-related pneumocystis carinii pneumonia. Chest 1990; 98: 1463-6

30. Fenwick JC, Dodek PM, Ronco JJ, Phang PT, Wiggs B, Russell JA. Increased concentrations of plasma lactate predict pathological dependence of oxygen consumption on oxygen delivery in patients with adult respiratory distress syndrome. J Crit Care 1990; 5: 81-7

31. Ronco JJ, Phang PT, Walley KR, Wiggs B, Fenwick JC, Russel JA. Oxygen consumption is independent of changes in oxygen delivery in severe adult respiratory distress syndrome. Am Rev Respir Dis 1991; 143: 1267-73

32. Shah DM, Gottlieb ME, Rahm RL, Stratton HH, Barie PS, Paloski WH, Newell JC. Failure of red blood cell transfusion to increase oxygen transport or mixed venous PO2 in injured patients. J Trauma 1982; 22: 741-6

33. Steffes CP, Bender JS, Levison MA. Blood transfusion and oxygen consumption in surgical sepsis. Crit Care Med 1991; 19: 512-7

34. Babineau TJ, Dzik WH, Borlase BC, Baxter JK, Bistrian BR, Benotti PN. Reevaluation of current transfusion practices in patients in surgical intensive care units. Am J Surg 1992; 164: 22-5

35. Casutt M, Seifert B, Pasch T, Schmid ER, Turina MI, Spahn DR. Factors influencing the individual effects of blood transfusions on oxygen delivery and oxygen consumption. Crit Care Med 1999; 27: 2194-200

36. Messmer K. Blood rheology factors and capillary blood flow, tissue oxygen utilization. Edited by Gutierrez G, Vincent J-L. Berlin, Heidelberg, New-York, Springer-Verlag, 1991, pp 103-13

37. Lipowsky HH, Firrel JC. Microvascular hemodynamics during systemic hemodilution and hemoconcentration. Am J Physiol 1986; 250: H908-H922

38. Vicaut E, Stucker O, Teisseire B, Duvelleroy M. Effects of changes in systemic hematocrit on the microcirculation in rat cremaster muscle. Int J Microcirc Clin Exp 1987; 6: 225-35

39. Stratton HH, Feustel PJ, Newell JC. Regression of calculated variables in the presence of shared measurement error. J Appl Physiol 1987; 62: 2083-93

40. Fitzgerald RD, Martin CM, Dietz GE, Doig GS, Potter RF, Sibbald WJ. Transfusing red blood cells stored in citrate phosphate dextrose adenine-1 for 28 days fails to improve tissue oxygenation in rats. Crit Care Med 1997; 25: 726-32

41. Sielenkämper AW, Chin-Yee IH, Martin CM, Sibbald WJ. Diaspirin crosslinked hemoglobin improves systemic oxygen uptake in oxygen supply-dependent septic rats. Am J Respir Crit Care Med 1997; 156: 1066-72

42. Haraldin AR, Weed RI, Reed CF. Changes in physical properties of stored erythrocytes. Transfusion 1969; 9: 229-35

43. Argawal JB, Paltoo R, Palmer WH. Relative viscosity of blood at varying hematocrits in pulmonary circulation. J Appl Physiol 1970; 29: 866-71

44. Friedlander MH, Simon R, Machiedo GW. The relationship of packed cell transfusion to red blood cell deformability in systemic inflammatory response syndrome patients. Shock 1998; 9: 84-8

45. Machiedo GW, Powell RJ, Rush BF, Swislocki NI, Dikdan G. The incidence of decreased red blood cell deformability in sepsis and the association with oxygen free radical damage and multiple-system organ failure. Arch Surg 1989; 124: 1386-9

46. Van der Linden P, De Hert S, Bélisle S, De Groote F, Mathieu N, D'Eugenio S, Julien V, Huynh C, Melot C. Comparative effects of red blood cell transfusion and increasing blood flow on tissue oxygenation in oxygen supply-dependent conditions. Am J Respir Crit Care Med 2001; 163: 1605-8

47. Hébert PC, Wells G, Blajchman MA, Marshall J, Martin C, Pagliarello G, Tweeddale MG, Schweitzer I, Yetisir E. A multicenter randomized controlled clinical trial of transfusion requirements in critical Care. N Engl J Med 1999; 340: 409-17

Plasma substitutes

3. Plasma substitutes

3.1. Crystalloids/Hypertonic solutions

3.1.1. Introduction

Crystalloids are commonly used in clinical practice to substitute fluid derangements in connection with surgical procedures or in the treatment of critically ill patients. It is well known that the general response of the body to trauma and blood loss is a neuroendocrine activation resulting in internal changes of the fluid homeostasis between the different fluid spaces of the body (1). The main components of this endogenous plasma volume supporting defence mechanism are resetting of the pre- to postcapillary resistance ratio, and a glucose-osmotic transcapillary refill process, whereby in the adult individual about 1.0 L of fluid can be transferred into the intravascular compartment from the intracellular and interstitial spaces. At the same time increased trauma-induced activation of the cascade systems, evoking a systemic inflammatory response syndrome (SIRS), may influence endothelial cell barrier function and capillary permeability and induce additional internal fluid fluxes into traumatised tissues (wounds edema) and into organs, the function of which is disturbed (e.g. paralytic intestine). Such fluid fluxes have been referred to as third space losses (2).

On the basis of the above aspects Shires and co-workers (2), probably being the most influential pro-crystalloid advocators since the 1960s, have suggested that in order to achieve normovolemia and hemodynamic stability, and to re-establish fluid homeostasis in surgical patients or trauma victims, it is necessary at the fluid resuscitation not only to consider direct blood losses but also all the internal compensatory fluid fluxes (2). Since extravascular fluids are primarily involved in these endogenous physiological fluid fluxes in response to trauma and to hypovolemia, it was suggested that crystalloid rather than a colloid resuscitation fluid should be chosen to re-establish internal fluid homeostasis. Such a hypothesis is supported by recent meta-analytic studies (3,4) suggesting that crystalloids may be superior in the treatment of critically ill patients with increased capillary permeability. However, the relevance of conclusions

based on meta-analysis of old studies for present clinical practice may be questioned (5).

3.1.2. Isotonic crystalloid solutions

3.1.2.1. General aspects on composition

Isotonic crystalloid solutions with varying electrolyte composition and sometimes also including glucose, lactate or acetate are available on the market. Several of these fluids have an electrolyte composition different from that of blood plasma. Such fluids are suitable for perioperative use to provide rehydration following preoperative fluid restriction and to substitute for basal fluid requirements. "Balanced" Ringer's type of solution is most commonly used for plasma volume support, but still reports on experiences from the use of physiological saline are common in the medical literature (6,7).

Saline 0.9 % is considered physiological, mainly from osmolality point of view, and it is sometimes used as a plasma volume substitute for extensive fluid resuscitation in connection with critical illness or in the perioperative period. The overall experience is that such a routine may affect the strong ion difference and thereby include a risk of development of clinically relevant hyperchloremic acidosis (6). It should also be remembered that many of the available colloids are based on isotonic saline. Therefore, the combination of 0.9 % saline and such an isotonic-saline-based colloid in the fluid resuscitation will further enhance the chloride load and increase the risk of overt hyperchloremic acidosis. Additional adverse effects on body homeostasis, in addition to acidosis, that have been observed following massive 0.9 % physiological saline fluid resuscitation are disturbed hemostasis and increased perioperative blood loss (6,7). Although such changes may not affect overall clinical outcome of surgical patients, still the problems can be avoided by the use Ringer's type of solutions with a balanced electrolyte composition (7). Ringer's type of solution for plasma volume support usually contains about 110 mMol/L of Cl^- as compared to 154 mMol/L of Cl^- in normal saline.

Crystalloids having a Ringer's fluid type of electrolyte composition, i.e. an electrolyte composition grossly similar to that of plasma, are the most suitable ones for plasma volume support. Usually such fluids have a "buffering capacity" which is dependent on their content of either lactate or acetate (1,8). When the lactate or acetate ions are metabolised by tissue cells, bicarbonate will be produced and a buffer effect is thereby achieved. Although lactate containing Ringer's type of solutions are most commonly used, the choice of acetate containing Ringer's solutions may be more advantageous since the capacity of the body to metabolise lactate may be reduced in case of severely disturbed organ perfusion, as seen in the connection with critical shock and trauma conditions (1,8). In such situations the infusion of a lactate containing solution may aggravate already existing lactic acidosis since the metabolic capacity of the two main lactate-clearing organs, the liver and the kidney, may be critically disturbed. Acetate, on the other hand, can be metabolised by most tissue cells of the body. Therefore, Ringer's acetate but not Ringer's lactate type of solutions will maintain a considerable buffer capacity also when used for fluid resuscitation of severe shock conditions.

3.1.2.2. Advantages of isotonic crystalloid resuscitation fluids

The use of isotonic crystalloids in clinical fluid resuscitation includes advantages as well as disadvantages (Table 3.1). Among the advantages of Ringer's type of crystalloid solutions, in addition to above considered balanced electrolyte composition and buffering capacity, are absence of risk of adverse anaphylactoid type of reactions and minimal influences on hemostasis other than effects caused by the hemodilution *per se*.

However, Ruttmann *et al* (9) have reported that dilution of blood *in vitro* as well as *in vivo* with crystalloid will increase whole blood coagulation (as measured by thrombelastography, TEG). It was observed that after initial crystalloid fluid load coagulation was enhanced. Therefore, it was concluded that perioperative coagulation mechanisms are triggered by rapid crystalloid hemodilution which seems to exert a procoagulant effect, possibly by enhancement of thrombin formation. Circulating concentrations of antithrombin III have been found more depleted than could be explained

by hemodilution alone (9). The clinical importance of these *in vitro* TEG-measured alterations in blood coagulation induced by saline or Ringer's is not fully understood and therefore disputed.

Advantages	Disadvantages
• Balanced electrolyte composition	• Poor plasma volume support
• Buffering capacity, lactate/acetate	• Large quantities needed
• No risk of adverse reactions	• Reduced plasma COP
• No disturbance of hemostasis	• Risk of overhydration
• Promoting diuresis	• Risk of edema formation
• Inexpensive	• Risk of hypothermia

Table 3.1: Advantages/disadvantages of crystalloid fluid resuscitation (1,8). COP: colloid osmotic pressure.

Additional beneficial clinical characteristics of crystalloids are diuresis promoting effects (Table 3.1). Furthermore, the low cost of crystalloid solutions, as compared to colloids, is often considered advantageous but the prerequisite for such a factor being a true clinical advantage is that no other adverse effects are induced that could affect clinical outcome and thereby the cost factor.

3.1.2.3. Disadvantages of crystalloid resuscitation fluids

Disadvantages associated with the use of crystalloid for plasma volume support are summarized in Table 3.1.

■ Excessive tissue hydration/edema formation

Salt solutions will freely cross capillary membranes and equilibrate within the whole extracellular compartment. Within 20-30 min 75-80 % of the infused volume will lodge mainly in the interstitial fluid space (1,8). In the hypovolemic patient infusion of a relatively large volume of fluid, about 3 to 4 or even up to 5 times the estimated intravascular volume deficit, is necessary in order to achieve normovolemia and hemodynamic stability. At the same time plasma colloid osmotic pressure (COP) will be reduced and a new Starling equilibrium for transcapillary fluid exchange will be established between the intravascular and the interstitial compartments. Therefore, it is obvious that the low plasma volume expending capacity of crystalloids, necessitating infusion of large volume of fluid, is associated with a risk of excessive tissue hydration and the development of tissue edema at crystalloid fluid resuscitation (1,8). Although it is usually claimed that extravascular fluid will accumulate mainly in tissues with a high compliance such as skin and connective tissue, experimental studies indicate that the fluid content is also increased in vital organs, e.g. in the lungs and the gastrointestinal tract (1,8).

The practical clinical experience is that a significant weight gain at the fluid resuscitation may be associated with increased need of respiratory treatment, impaired wound healing, and prolonged ICU stay. Such a fluid overload may disturb the recovery process after surgery and trauma, particularly in elderly patients with reduced functional capacity of vital organs, including the cardiovascular and respiratory systems. Arieff (10) has retrospectively assessed the possible cause of fatal postoperative pulmonary edema. He found that patients suffering such a complication had a net fluid retention of at least 67 mL/kg in the initial 24 postoperative hours. Of the 13 patients facing mortality, 10 were generally healthy while only 3 had serious associated disease prior to surgery and fluid resuscitation. Autopsy revealed pulmonary edema with no other possible cause of death. In the clinic no predictive warning signs of a fluid overload were found and the most frequent clinical presentation was cardiorespiratory arrest. Positive fluid balance (exceeding 4 L) may also be a strong risk factor for postoperative pulmonary complications and in-hospital mortality in connection with elective pneumonectomy. The problem of extravascular fluid accumulation after crystalloid volume loading seems even more critical for trauma patients suffering head injury. Furthermore, initial resuscitation with large quantities of crystalloid may induce late adverse effects on cardiorespiratory function, seen as a "third-day" transient circulatory overload caused by a redistribution of tissue edema (1,8). Therefore, it seems obvious that excessive crystalloid fluid resuscitation is associated with considerable risk of increased morbidity and even mortality.

Clinical studies indicate that the formation of interstitial edema can be prevented by avoiding COP decreases. Lang et al (11) have reported perioperative fluid resuscitation with lactated Ringer's solution in major abdominal surgery to cause a reduction of tissue oxygen tension in the deltoid muscle of about 23 % while 6 % HES (130 kD/0.4) was found to improve skeletal muscle oxygenation by up to 59 % from the baseline level. As pointed out by these authors, fluid administration should not only stabilize macrohemodynamics but also have beneficial effects on microcirculation and tissue oxygenation. Similar experiences have been reported by Prien et al (12). They found that formation of intestinal edema could be prevented during lengthy gastrointestinal surgery by avoiding COP decreases.

■ Hypothermia

Infusion of large quantities of cold fluids may induce hypothermia which is known to be associated with risk of cardiac arrhythmias, impaired tissue perfusion, metabolic disturbances, and coagulopathy (13). Many of the coagulation reactions occur insufficiently at a temperature below 37°C and platelet function is impaired. Hypothermia will furthermore reduce the hepatic synthesis of coagulation factors. Since large volume of crystalloid is needed in the resuscitation of severe hypovolemia, it is of importance to prevent such deleterious temperature dependent effects by proper warming of intravenously administered fluids. Thereby the risk of bleeding complications and excessive blood losses may be attenuated.

The temperature of the infused fluid has been reported also to affect the overall distribution of the fluid between the intra- and extravascular spaces and furthermore to influence transcapillary filtration rate as well as atrial natriuretic factor production and diuresis (14). In healthy volunteers infusion of cold (18°C) Ringer's acetate was found to increase blood pressure in response to the volume load and to enhance atrial natriuretic factor production whereby diuresis was promoted. Heart rate reduction was also observed which could be caused by the decrease in temperature of the blood returning to the heart. Infusion of warm (36°C) Ringer's acetate, on the other hand, was shown not to influence blood pressure but instead to induce peripheral vasodilation, increased skin temperature, and capillary leakage (14). The increased capillary filtration of fluid into the interstitial space was considered to reduce interstitial COP and promote edema formation. The clinical relevance of these changes observed in healthy volunteers for the response pattern of critically ill, hypovolemic patients is not known. The general clinical concept to be favoured, however, is that intravenously administered fluids should be warmed, especially if massive volume therapy is needed, unless body temperature of the fluid recipient is increased in response to fever caused by infectious complications/septic states.

The technical requirements for equipment for optimal warming during fluid replacement have been well characterized but although the optimal infusate temperature should be close to 37°C it may still be difficult to reach this optimal temperature level even with modern fluid warmers during massive transfusions.

3.1.3. Hypertonic solutions

Hypertonic saline (HS) resuscitation in hypovolemic shock is considered advantageous since HS has been shown experimentally as well as clinically to increase systemic blood pressure, cardiac output, peripheral tissue perfusion, and survival rates (15-18). Most commonly a 7.5 % NaCl (2,400 mosmol/l) solution (with or with colloid) is used.

	HyperHaes™ (Fresenius, Germany)	RescueFlow™ (BioPhausia, Sweden)
Electrolyte concentration	7.2 % NaCl	7.5 % NaCl
Sodium	1,232 mmol/l	1,283 mmol/l
Theoretical osmolarity	2,464 mosmol/l	2,567 mosmol/l
Colloid	hydroxyethyl starch	dextran
Colloid concentration	6 %	6 %
Mean molecular weight (kD)	200	70
Indication	severe volume deficit	severe volume deficit

Table 3.2: Characteristics of hypertonic-colloid solutions.

The volume infused in the treatment of hypovolemia is small, usually about 4 mL/kg body weight, i.e. a small-volume resuscitation principle bases on rapid infusion of approximately 250 mL in an adult individual. This small-volume principle should be compared to the large fluid volume requirements of about 4 to 5 times the blood volume deficit that have to be infused when isotonic crystalloid solutions are used in the treatment of hypovolemia and shock.

3.1.3.1. Hypertonic solutions – physiological responses

The general mechanisms of action of HS solutions are summarized in Table 3.3. The central hemodynamic support induced by HS is the result of rapid mobilization of fluid from the extra- and intracellular compartments into the vascular compartment.

Fluid redistribution
• increased intravascular volume
- hemodilution
- reduced blood viscosity
- increased venous return
- increased preload
- increased cardiac output
Vasodilation
• reduced afterload
- improved regional blood flow
- reduced cardiac work
Cellular shrinkage
• improved capillary blood flow
• reduced tissue edema
Direct effects on cell function
• central sympathetic activation
• cellular functional alterations

Table 3.3: Physiological responses to hypertonic saline (HS) infusion.

Studies assessing the relative importance of osmolarity as compared to ionic composition of hypertonic solutions in shock treatment clearly demonstrate an important functional role of concentrated sodium ions. Electrolyte solutions based on cations other than sodium or anions other than chloride do not reverse hemorrhagic shock and improve survival rates as efficiently as hypertonic sodium chloride (15-18). The importance of the sodium ion as compared to osmolarity per se for the efficacy of hypertonic fluid therapy in shock is well documented and a high plasma sodium level seems essential for survival.

The hemodilution that follows the HS-induced dynamic fluid redistribution offers hemorheological advantages. Blood flow through the terminal vascular bed is improved and venous return is enhanced. There is an efficient restitution of organ perfusion following HS infusion, especially if a hypertonic-hyperoncotic fluid combination rather than HS alone is chosen. The beneficial effects of HS on microvascular blood flow are probably multifactorial. A deswelling of blood cells and vascular endothelial cells will occur following infusion of HS in addition to the direct vasodilatory effects of HS (Table 3.3).

It has been well documented that treatment of hypovolemic conditions with HS solutions improves cardiac output. The direct effects of HS on myocardial performance may, however, be slightly depressant rather than stimulatory. Physiological mechanisms other than direct inotropic myocardial cell effects may be partly responsible for the cardiovascular stimulatory actions of HS treatment. Central sympathetic activity seems enhanced by increased sodium levels. HS therapy also promotes diuresis which may be of importance for prevention of renal dysfunction in the trauma patient.

There are several potential disadvantages of HS therapy. In addition to local pain at the site of infusion and transient negative effects on cardiac function, a risk of increased bleeding due to vasodilatory effects has been suggested (15-18). Since HS (7.5 % NaCl) resuscitation will provide a rather high chloride load in spite of the usually practiced small volume principle (4 mL/kg b.w.), it may include a risk of inducing transient hyperchloremic acidosis.

3.1.3.2. Hypertonic solutions in shock and trauma resuscitation

Prehospital or initial intrahospital small volume resuscitation in hypovolemic shock seems advantageous since HS has been shown experimentally as well as clinically to increase systemic blood pressure, cardiac output, peripheral tissue perfusion, and survival rates (15-17). Survival data of severely injured patients similarly favour treatment regimens combining hypertonic and hyperoncotic fluid components (15). Meta-analysis of the efficacy of hypertonic 7.5 % saline in combination with colloid in treating trauma indicates that the HS-colloid combination is superior to the conventional volume replacement strategy (15).

With respect to the actual data base of clinical trials HS resuscitation seems to be superior to conventional volume therapy with regard to faster normalization of microvascular perfusion during shock phases and early resumption of organ function. Patients with head trauma in association with systemic hypotension appear to benefit in particular (15-17). According to Kreimeier and Messmer (17) small-volume resuscitation by means of hypertonic NaCl/colloid solutions stands for one of the most innovative concepts for primary resuscitation from trauma and shock established in the past decade. Also, for treatment of patients with sepsis it seems increasingly obvious from available data that HS may include potential benefits (18). HS treatment will moderate a number of sepsis-induced pathophysiological disturbances such as tissue hypoperfusion, decreased oxygen consumption, endothelial cell dysfunction, cardiac depression, and the presence of a broad array of proinflammatory cytokines and various oxidant species (18). Although the goals of research in the fields of shock, trauma and sepsis resuscitation are to identify reliable therapies to prevent ischemia and inflammation, and to reduce mortality, still, however, the overall clinical experience with HS-solutions is somewhat limited and the final role of small-volume HS in shock and trauma resuscitation needs further documentation (15-18).

3.1.3.3. Hypertonic solutions in routine surgery

Potential advantages of perioperative HS fluid therapy in connection with certain surgical procedures and in the intensive care setting have become more and more obvious in recent years (17,18). HS fluid therapy may be of specific advantage in situations in which excess free water administration is to be avoided but the intravascular volume needs correction. This applies to aortic surgery, cardiac surgery as well as other types of surgery including plasma volume support in connection with regional (spinal) anesthesia (17,19,20).

In connection with both elective and emergency abdominal aortic aneurysm repair infusion of HS in combination with colloid over 20 minutes has been shown to improve hemodynamic parameters and result in a less positive overall fluid balance, thus decreasing the likelihood of edema formation (17). Since a largely positive perioperative fluid balance may put the patients at risk of developing left ventricular failure and increased morbidity HS fluid therapy seems advantageous to use in aortic aneurysm surgery.

In connection with cardiac surgery pre-, intra- and postoperative HS infusion has been shown to be associated with beneficial effects (19). Extracorporeal circulation is known to induce increased capillary permeability with fluid leakage into the interstitial space, resulting in positive fluid balance and intravascular hypovolemia. HS and colloid infused after coronary artery surgery has been found to mobilize such fluid excess, improve cardiorespiratory functions (increase cardiac output, reduce intrapulmonary venous admixture, improve PaO_2), and increase diuresis (19).

Prevention of hypotension during spinal anesthesia by using HS instead of isotonic Ringer's type of fluid preloading is an additional interesting approach (20). HS seems effective at infusion of small doses (1.6 mL/kg) by which extracellular water, plasma volume and cardiac output are increased and hemodynamic stability maintained during spinal anesthesia. Therefore, HS seems a valuable alternative for fluid preloading before spinal anesthesia in situations where excess free water administration is not desired.

■ **Concerns associated with the use of HS in normovolemic/awake individuals**

The use of HS in the perioperative setting, especially in the awake and in the normovolemic patient, may include some specific concerns.

The high osmolality of about 2,400 mosmol/kg H_2O and may induce local inflammatory responses at the site of infusion. Therefore, it is not surprising that HS infusion has been reported to be associated with local sensations of heat and compression during the ongoing infusion (20). However, the unpleasant sensations seem to disappear immediately after the completion of the HS infusion. Since usually a small volume (about 4 mL/kg b.w.) of HS is infused, it appears that these local adverse effects of HS fluid therapy are rather mild and seem well tolerated (19). Rather rapid i.v. infusion of HS (7.5 % NaCl + 6 % DEX 70, HSD) at a dosage of 4 mL/kg b.w. within 10 min has, in addition to local sensations, been reported also to cause a sensation of heat starting in the upper part of thorax and spreading upwards to the throat, face, and head (21). Slight headache for a few minutes or euphoric feelings may ensue. Such unpleasant transitory sensations of headache and/or heat in the thorax following infusion of HSD seem more pronounced in normovolemic than in hypovolemic individuals.

The mobilization of fluid from the intracellular into the intravascular compartment in a normovolemic individual includes a potential risk of transiently increased intravascular volume load. Therefore, in spite of the small volume infused there can be a pronounced hemodynamic response resulting in a markedly increased blood pressure and increased heart rate (21). Such a response pattern may be hazardous for a patient with critical cardiovascular disease and could include a risk of myocardial ischemia and cardiac failure. Thus, it is of importance to monitor closely the hemodynamic effects of the HS fluid load and also to have strict blood pressure criteria for starting HS therapy to resuscitate trauma patients.

Transient hypotension is an additional risk factor associated with the infusion of HS. The reasons of such a response may be acute reduction in systemic vascular resistance and negative effects on myocardial function in addition to acute volume overload in patients with latent or manifest cardiac failure at too vigorous volume load (16,17,21). Kien and coworkers (22) have suggested that the acute hypotension caused by rapid infusion of HS may not be mediated by cardiac depression but rather by a marked decrease in total peripheral vascular resistance. Studies of the effects of HS on the isolated denervated, ischemic as well as non-ischemic heart, however, indicate transient direct myocardial depressant effects of HS-infusion (23). Therefore, a risk of initial transient hypotension due to myocardial depression as well as reduced total peripheral resistance must be taken into account in association with HS-based fluid resuscitation, especially in case of rapid intravenous infusion.

3.1.4. Conclusions

Crystalloids are commonly used for correction of extravasacular fluid derangements but infusion of large volumes for correction of major intravascular volume deficits includes a risk of tissue overhydration, edema formation, and organ dysfunction unless combined with colloid (24). All types of intravenous fluids - crystalloids as well as colloids - may induce adverse reactions in case of improper use or presence of patient associated specific risk factors. Systemic adverse responses to fluid therapy caused by too rapid infusion or excessive fluid administration resulting in hypervolemia, circulatory overload, or, in case of fluid therapy with mainly crystalloids, formation of tissue edema or development of hyperchloremic acidosis, can be avoided by proper choice of type of fluid and by adequate monitoring of the fluid therapy. Although small-volume resuscitation by using hypertonic NaCl solutions, usually in combination with a colloid, is an innovative concept for primary resuscitation from trauma and shock as well as in the perioperative or ICU setting, the overall clinical experience with HS-solutions is somewhat limited and further documentation is needed before the clinical potential of small-volume HS resuscitation can be fully established.

3.1.5. References

1. Haljamäe H. Use of fluids in trauma. Int J Intensive Care 1999; 6: 20-30.

2. Shires GT, Barber AE, Illner HP. Current status of resuscitation: solutions including hypertonic saline. Adv Surg. 1995; 28: 133-170.

3. Schierhout G, Roberts I. Fluid resuscitation with colloid or crystalloid solutions in critically ill patients: a systematic review of randomised trials. BMJ 1998; 316: 961-964.

4. Choi PT, Yip G, Quinonez LG, Cook DJ. Crystalloids vs. colloids in fluid resuscitation: a systematic review. Crit Care Med 1999; 27: 200-210.

5. Webb AR. Crystalloid or colloid for resuscitation. Are we any the wiser? Crit Care 1999; 3: R25-R28.

6. Stephens RC, Mythen MG. Saline based fluids can cause a significant acidosis that may be clinically relevant. Crit Care Med 2000; 28: 3375-3377.

7. Waters JH, Gottlieb A, Schoenwald P, Popovich MJ, Sprung J, Nelson DR. Normal saline versus lactated Ringer's solution for intraoperative fluid management in patients undergoing abdominal aortic aneurysm repair: an outcome study. Anesth Analg 2001; 93: 817-822.

8. Haljamäe H. Crystalloids versus colloids: The controversy. In: NATA Textbook. R & J Éditions Médicale, Paris, 1999: 27-36.

9. Ruttmann TG, James MF, Finlayson J. Effects on coagulation of intravenous crystalloid or colloid in patients undergoing peripheral vascular surgery.Br J Anaesth 2002; 89:2 26-230.

10. Arieff AI. Fatal postoperative pulmonary edema: pathogenesis and literature review. Chest 1999; 115: 1371-1377.

11. Lang K, Boldt J, Suttner S, Haisch G. Colloids versus crystalloids and tissue oxygen tension in patients undergoing major abdominal surgery. Anesth Analg 2001; 93: 405-409.

12. Prien T, Backhaus N, Pelser F, Pircher W, Bünte H, Lawin P. Effects of intraoperative fluid administration and colloid osmotic pressure on the formation of intestinal edema during gastrointestinal surgery. J Clin Anesth 1990; 2: 317-323.

13. Rohrer MJ, Natale AM. Effect of hypothermia on the coagulation cascade. Crit Care Med 1992; 20: 1402-1405.

14. Tølløfsrud S, Bjerkelund CE, Kongsgaard U, Hall C, Noddeland H. Cold and warm infusion of Ringer's acetate in healthy volunteers: the effects on haemodynamic parameters, transcapillary fluid balance, diuresis and atrial peptides. Acta Anaesthesiol Scand 1993; 37: 768-773.

15. Wade CE, Kramer GC, Grady JJ, Fabian TC, Younes RN. Efficacy of hypertonic 7.5 % saline and 6 % dextran-70 in treating trauma: a meta-analysis of controlled clinical studies. Surgery. 1997; 122: 609-616.

16. Haljamäe H, McCunn M. Fluid resuscitation and circulatory support: Fluids – when, what, and how much? In: Prehospital Trauma Care. Eds: E. Søreide & CM Grande. Marcel Dekker Inc., New York, 2001, pp 299-322.

17. Kreimeier U, Messmer K. Small-volume resuscitation: from experimental evidence to clinical routine. Advantages and disadvantages of hypertonic solutions. Acta Anaesthesiol Scand 2002; 46: 625-638.

18. Oliveira RP, Velasco I, Soriano F, Friedman G. Clinical review: Hypertonic saline resuscitation in sepsis. Crit Care 2002; 6: 418-423.

19. Tølløfsrud S, Mathru M, Kramer GC. Hypertonic-hyperoncotic solutions in open-heart surgery. Perfusion 1998; 13: 289-296.

20. Järvelä K, Kööbi T, Kauppinen P, Kaukinen S. Effects of hypertonic 75 mg/ml (7.5 %) saline on extracellular water volume when used for preloading before spinal anaesthesia. Acta Anaesthesiol Scand 2001; 45: 776-781.

21. Tølløfsrud S, Tønnessen T, Skraastad O, Noddeland H. Hypertonic saline and dextran in normovolaemic and hypovolaemic healthy volunteers increases interstitial and intravascular fluid volumes. Acta Anaesthesiol Scand 1998; 42: 145-153.

22. Kien ND, Kramer GC, White DA. Acute hypotension caused by rapid hypertonic saline infusion in anesthetized dogs. Anesth Analg 1991; 73: 597-602.

23. Waagstein L, Haljamäe H, Ricksten S-E, Sahlman L. Effects of hypertonic saline on myocardial function and metabolism in non-ischemic and ischemic isolated working rat heart. Crit Care Med 1995; 23: 1890-1897.

24. Haljamäe H, Dahlqvist M, Walentin F. Artificial colloids in clinical practice: pros and cons. Baillière´s Clin Anaesthesiol 1997; 11: 49-79.

3.2. Albumin

3.2.1. Introduction

Historically, albumin is perhaps the best known and most extensively studied of all proteins. Hippocrates guessed it caused frothy urine in kidney failure. 'Albumen' (early German for protein), was recognised by Harvey as a constituent of serum in the seventeenth century. In the mid nineteenth century H.Ancell found 'albumen' in many other animal fluids e.g. chyle and lymph. By the early twentieth century, the protein composition of blood had been worked out by salt fractionation and crystallisation. Albumin became a single reproducible substance.

The use of albumin as a volume replacement fluid owes much to World War II. The tremendous shortage of blood for transfusion on the battlefield created a need for a stable blood plasma substitute. In 1940, it became evident that albumin may be better than whole plasma for infusion, because it was less antigenic, more stable in solution and less viscous. A team at the Harvard Medical School had developed a method of purifying albumin from bovine plasma, using a technique known as cold fractionation. Serum sickness was not known about in the 1940's, and it was only after several deaths in volunteers that the bovine program was stopped. Albumin was purified from human plasma in 1941. The most famous early use of human albumin was after the Pearl Harbor attack, when virtually the entire stock was given to seven patients with severe burns. All of them survived. This led to a huge expansion in albumin production and use during the war. Availability bred familiarity, and albumin became a common choice for volume replacement among surgeons and nutritionists after the war. Extensive research continues into the twenty-first century.

3.2.2. Anatomy and physiology of albumin

Albumin is the most plentiful soluble protein in all vertebrates. In humans, it accounts for 55-60 % of measured serum protein. The molecule consists of a single polypeptide chain of 585 amino acids, wrapped into a heart-shaped structure of three domains. However, in vivo it can vary shape and structure to fulfil its role as a transport and scavenging vehicle. In solution albumin appears ellipsoidal, which reduces viscosity, but it can easily return to its folded shape, trapping a wide range of substances within. Given the right environmental conditions, the 17 disulfide bridges holding the molecule together are breached, releasing the ligand at the relevant target site. An elegant and very efficient cargo transport system.

Vascular	• Maintenance of oncotic pressure • Microvascular integrity

Transport	• Hormones – steroids, thyroxine
	• Fatty acids
	• Bile salts
	• Bilirubin
	• Ca^{2+}, Mg^{2+} and other metals (copper, zinc)
	• Drugs
	  - warfarin
	  - diazepam

Metabolic	• Acid base balance • Antioxidant • Anticoagulant

Table 3.4: Functions of albumin.

Table 3.4 lists the many important functions of albumin in health. The principal function with regard to this chapter is that of its role in the maintenance of intravascular volume. It is responsible for 80 % of the normal colloid osmotic pressure in the bloodstream. Albumin has a relatively low molecular weight (66,500 Daltons) and a high intravascular concentration (40 g/L) compared with other plasma proteins. This produces significant colloidal activity. Activity is additionally enhanced by the many negative charges on the molecule. This is known as the Gibbs-Donnan effect. The strong negative charge attract positive ions, especially sodium (Na^+). Na^+ is the most abundant extracellular positive ion and is highly osmotically active, hence water is held in the vascular space.

Albumin does not remain exclusively within the vascular space. The serum concentration of albumin will depend on its synthesis, degradation and distribution between intravascular and extravascular compartments. Figure 3.1a illustrates this. The total body albumin pool is between 3.5 and 5.0 g/kg body weight. About 40 % of this is intravascular. The remaining 60 % is extravascular. Over two thirds of the extravascular albumin is exchangeable with the intravascular albumin (the exchangeable pool). Some albumin is tissue-bound and unavailable to the circulation (this is the remote pool). A very small amount is normally lost via the gut and kidneys. It is worth noting that half the extravascular pool is in the skin, which accounts for the large albumin losses seen in burns patients. In health the serum albumin concentration is maintained within a narrow range by close coupling of the rates of synthesis and degradation, and exchange between the compartments (see Figure 3.1b).

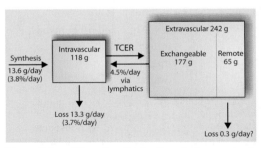

Figure 3.1a: Albumin distribution between body compartments. Values given are typical for a 70kg adult male.
TCER = trans-capillary escape rate - see Figure 3.1b. Albumin can freely cross into the extravascular space when the capillaries are not continuous. For instance, the liver and bone marrow have wide-open sinusoids between vascular and interstitial compartments. In the small intestine, pancreas and adrenal glands the capillaries are fenestrated, and the rate of exchange in these tissues depends on the permeability of the wall as well as hydrostatic and oncotic pressures on either

side of the wall. 50 % of the escaping albumin passes through the continuous capillaries, and this requires an active transport mechanism. Albumin binds to a surface receptor called albondin which mediates active endocytosis.

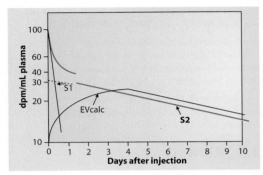

Figure 3.1b: Decay pattern of labelled albumin versus time after IV injection of a tracer dose of ^{125}I-labelled HSA (dark line).
There is a rapid phase of disappearance from the plasma over the first two days. This represents the transcapillary exchange rate (TCER) of 4.5 %/hour, giving a distribution half time ($t_{1/2\ dist}$) of about 15 hours - slope 1 (S1). Then there is a slower exponential decay representing the fractional degradation rate (FDR) of about 3.7 %/day, with an elimination half time ($t_{1/2\ elim}$) of about 19 days - slope 2 (S2). The FDR closely parallels the rate of synthesis in steady state (3.8 %/day). EVcalc is the calculated increase in extravascular labelled albumin concentration. Note that the activity of extravascular albumin is greater than intravascular albumin from about day 3 onwards. This suggests that degradation occurs directly from the vascular compartment - see Figure 3.1a (14).

Albumin is synthesised in the liver. About 12 to 25 g of albumin are made each day (1). The rate of synthesis varies with nutritional and disease states. However much of the liver's synthetic apparatus is already occupied by albumin synthesis, and the maximum rate is only 2.5 times normal. The process is summarised in Figure 3.2.

Albumin will only be synthesised in a suitable nutritional, hormonal and osmotic environment. The colloid osmotic pressure of the interstitial fluid bathing the hepatocyte is the most important regulator of albumin synthesis.

Hormones important for adequate synthesis include insulin, corticosteroids and growth hormone. Diabetic subjects have a decreased synthetic rate, which improves with insulin infusion (2).

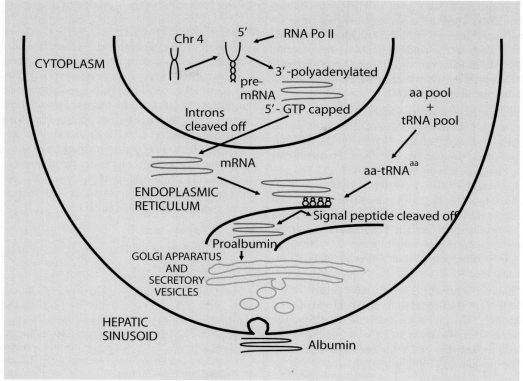

Figure 3.2: The synthetic pathway for albumin. Adapted from Moldave, K (1985) (16).
Synthesis consists of 3 processes:
(i) *Transcription:* The albumin gene lies on the long arm of chromosome 4. The DNA double helix uncoils with binding of regulatory proteins to nucleotide sequences called promoters or enhancers. RNA polymerase II can then bind to the the 5′ end of the DNA strand and copy it. The enlarging pre-mRNA has its 5′ end capped by GTP which protects it from RNase activity, and acts as a signal for ribosomal translation. When the 3′ end is reached, the mRNA chain is cleaved and poly-A-polymerase attaches 50-250 adenyl nucleotides (polyadenylation). Before leaving the nucleus, the introns are cleaved off and the 15 exons spliced together.
(ii) *Translation:* Ribosomes are responsible for translating the mRNA into an amino acid (aa) sequence. An initiation complex is formed, consisting of the mRNA, a ribosome, the relevant aa for each codon, and its tRNA. Elongation of the nascent chain depends on a cytoplasmic pool of relevant aa's, their tRNA's, and potential energy in the from of GTP or ATP. Terminator codons on the mRNA are recognised by the ribosomes which then cleave the final aa-tRNA bond. Multiple ribosomes can attach to one mRNA chain, producing multiple nascent albumin molecules. Such an aggregate of ribosomes on one mRNA is termed a polysome. Cytoplasmic polysomes contain 19 ribosomes per albumin mRNA. This equates to one ribosome every 34 codons, which is close to the maximum possible, testifying to the efficiency of albumin mRNA translation. Completion of one albumin chain takes about 1.5 to 2 minutes.
(iii) *Secretion:* Proteins destined for secretion are segregated from those destined for intracellular use by ribosomes. Free cytoplasmic ribosomes make intracellular proteins. Ribosomes bound to the endoplasmic reticulum (ER) are responsible for making proteins destined for secretion. We now know that this is the job of the signal peptide, the first 18-20 aa residues of the nascent chain. A signal recognition particle (SRP) binds both the signal peptide and a docking receptor on the ER. As the nascent chain elongates, the SRP is removed, the chain is transferred into the ER and the ribosome attaches to a specific receptor on the ER. The signal peptide is cleaved off the chain as it emerges from the luminal surface. The nascent chain still has a 6-residue propeptide at the front, and the molecule is now called proalbumin. This may have a role in directing the protein through the rER cisternae to the sER, the Golgi complex and into secretory vesicles. It is cleaved away at some point, probably in the secretory vesicle.

Corticosteroids have complex effects on albumin synthesis. There is increased albumin synthesis with combinations of steroids and insulin, and steroids with amino acids (1,3). However, steroids also increase albumin catabolism. Growth hormone has been shown to stimulate gene transcription in cultured hepatocytes (4).

Nutritional intake is important in regulating albumin synthesis, more so than for other hepatic proteins (1). Fasting reduces albumin production, but specifically omitting protein from the diet causes an even greater reduction in synthesis (5). The early effects of protein deprivation can be rapidly reversed by re-feeding with amino acids, but protein deprivation for a longer time leads to a 50-60 % decrease in synthetic activity. Calories are important, however and energy, rather than amino acid supply, may be more important under normal circumstances (6).

Albumin is broken down in most organs of the body. Half the degradation occurs in muscle and skin (7). The liver is responsible for only 15 %. The kidneys degrade about 10 %, while another 10 % leaks through the wall of the gastrointestinal tract. The breakdown of albumin involves uptake of the protein into endocytotic vesicles within cells of the relevant organs. The final breakdown products are free amino acids which are then available for protein synthesis.

Given the many functions of albumin in health, one might anticipate that a reduction in serum albumin in critical illness, trauma and other disease states should be treated by albumin infusion. However, there is no evidence to show a benefit in treating hypoalbuminemia under these conditions. It has been recently suggested by a meta-analysis that the use of albumin for plasma substitution may actually be harmful (8). This meta-analysis examined albumin use across a wide series of studies, looking at different population groups, and varied treatment regimes. The general consensus of current opinion is that properly conducted randomised controlled trials are required before any conclusions can be drawn. Albumin may be neither better nor worse as compared with other colloid therapies.

Critical illness and the activity of albumin

▶ Distribution of albumin

The distribution of albumin between intravascular and extravascular compartments in critical illness is altered. This is related to an increase in capillary leakage which occurs in sepsis (9), and after major surgical stress (10,11). The trans-capillary escape rate of albumin increases by up to 300 % in patients with septic shock, and by 100 % after cardiac surgery (9). There is no complementary increase in lymphatic return of this albumin to the intravascular space (11). Sequestration of albumin may occur into non-exchangeable areas such as wound, intestinal and extra-abdominal sites (12).

▶ Synthesis of albumin

The rate of albumin synthesis may be significantly altered in the critically ill (13). In the acute response to trauma, inflammation or sepsis there is increased synthesis of positive acute-phase proteins such as C-reactive protein (CRP), and a decreased synthesis of albumin. A sustained inflammatory response in critical illness may lead to prolonged inhibition of albumin synthesis.

▶ Breakdown of albumin

Catabolism of albumin may also be altered. Normally the rates of synthesis and degradation of albumin are equal. In critical illness this relationship is disrupted. Some studies show that there is an increase in breakdown of albumin. Others suggest that tissue trapping of albumin may reduce its availability for degradation.

▶ Structural changes in albumin

Further evidence reveals that many diseases are accompanied by conformational changes in the albumin molecule, despite little or no change in its concentration. This may contribute to changes in albumin function and rates of albumin breakdown.

Some people survive with virtually no circulating albumin. This interesting condition, analbuminemia, is due to a genetic mutation resulting in serum albumin levels of less than or equal to 1g/dL. Individuals with this condition are not usually diagnosed until early adulthood. The clinical manifestations are peripheral edema, a lipodystrophy giving lower limb obesity; fatigue; and hyperlipidemia, but without resultant atherosclerosis. Hemodynamic changes are minimal. There is a reduction in colloid oncotic pressure (COP) (16 mmHg versus 25) and a reduction in arterial pressure which leads to an increase in renin and aldosterone levels. The body seems to compensate by slowing the degradation rate of the small amount of albumin present.

3.2.3. Albumin solutions

There are two categories of albumin products: plasma protein fraction (PPF) and human albumin solution (HAS). The former has a higher yield, but a minimum albumin purity of only 85 %, which falls short by today's standards. HAS is purified using a less efficient process, but the purity of the product and consequent safety ensure its value. There are essentially two purification processes: cold fractionation, and chromatographic separation. The former has remained largely unaltered since 1946, and with minor modification is still in widespread use. Chromatographic purification was first offered as an alternative in the early 1980's. The process may be less damaging to the molecule, results in lower aggregate concentrations, will give a higher yield, and is probably cheaper. However, the equipment needed is not cheap, and until recently has been in short supply.

The latest manufacturing advance concerns the development of synthetic albumin via recombinant DNA.

Manufacture of albumin is from pooled human plasma using multiple sources, often imported from different countries. The emphasis is on eliminating impurities that may be associated with side-effects. For instance, hypotension after rapid infusion of early solutions was attributed to a high content of pre-kallikrein activator (PKA) (14). This causes an increase in circulating levels of bradykinin, a potent vasodilator. Aluminium contamination leads to accumulation of this metal in patients with poor kidney function, and in neonates. Trace proteins, if not removed, could result in aggregation during the pasteurisation of albumin solutions.

Lack of disease transmission is an important goal. The safety of albumin solutions over the last half-century is impressive. Solutions are pasteurised at 60°C for 10 hours. It has been shown that this will kill a range of viruses including Hepatitis A, B and C and HIV. This testifies to the robustness of the molecule, though stabilizers such as sodium caprylate are required to ensure the protein is not denatured. The latest scare concerns prion disease transmission. As yet we are not able to quantify this risk.

Adverse reactions may occur to albumin administration, including anaphylactoid reactions. A series of reported adverse reactions in 1990 suggested an incidence of 1 per 6,600 infusions. More recently spontaneous incident reporting has suggested that the incidence may be as low as 1 per 17,200 for 4.5 % albumin and 1 per 78,200 infusions for 20 % albumin (15). None of these reactions were fatal. It is accepted that spontaneous reporting will generally underestimate the true incidence.

3.2.4. Use of albumin

Currently albumin is rarely used for plasma substitution. Certainly hypoalbuminemia per se is not an indication for albumin infusion. Historically albumin has been used for plasma expansion because of its availability when there were few, if any, synthetic alternatives. At present, the use of albumin is restricted to patients with acute fulminant liver injury or after abdominal paracentesis for ascites. Animal experiments suggest that albumin may be superior to other plasma expanders in terms of liver cell recovery and renin/angiotensin system changes. Advocates of the use of albumin will argue its superiority over other colloids on the basis of its side-effect profile. It is thought to have a less deleterious effect on coagulation, does not have an upper limit on daily dosage and is not associated with the pruritus occasionally seen with the starches. Opposition is based largely on its high cost as compared with gelatins/starches. Albumin may be as much as ten times the cost of gelatins, and five times that of equivalent starches. Furthermore, there is a lack of evidence to suggest that albumin offers a survival advantage or any other improvement in outcome measures in critical care medicine.

3.2.5. How to give albumin

■ 4.5 % - 5 % Albumin - isotonic

Close monitoring of the patient's hemodynamic status is usually required when considering colloidal therapy, at a minimum, blood pressure, pulse rate and urine output. If the patient is unstable, then invasive arterial central venous monitoring may be required. This is usually done on an intensive care unit.

If albumin is selected as the colloid of choice, administration is independent of the serum albumin concentration.

If the patient is hypotensive (e.g. systolic blood pressure – SBP < 100 mmHg), tachycardic (e.g. pulse rate – PR > 100 beats/min), and oliguric (urine output – UOP < 0.5 mL/kg/hour), give a bolus of 100 – 250 mL isotonic albumin and assess the response. If a central venous pressure (CVP) line is in-situ, a useful guide to adequacy of plasma volume is maintenance of the increased pressure from the fluid bolus after 15 minutes. If the pressure falls within that time, then further fluid boluses may be required.

■ 20 % - 25 % Albumin – hypertonic

In patients with low plasma volume and high extravascular water, e.g. in hepatic cirrhosis, 20 % albumin solution is still used as a plasma expander. 100 mL will produce a volume expansion equivalent to 500 mL plasma, providing the patient does not have capillary leak syndrome.

In replacement of plasma volume during paracentesis, 100 mL of 20 % albumin can be given after drainage of a certain volume of ascites, e.g. 3 L. Central venous pressure monitoring is recommended, and fluid replacement adjusted accordingly.

Care should be taken to avoid over-expansion of the plasma volume, especially in patients with cardio-respiratory disease.

There is no evidence that giving albumin to correct hypoalbuminemia improves patient outcome.

3.2.6. Summary

- Albumin is abundant and multi-functional in vivo.
- Albumin has altered kinetics in disease states.
- Hypoalbuminemia is associated with reduced physiological function.
- There is no evidence that correcting hypoalbuniemia by giving albumin is beneficial.
- There is no proven benefit of albumin over other colloid therapies.
- Albumin is expensive compared to other plasma expanders.

- Albumin is still used for the treatment of plasma volume depletion associated with acute hepatic failure, and after paracentesis (drainage of ascites).

3.2.7. Conclusion

Historically albumin was revolutionary as a volume replacement therapy. It opened the door to the development of effective plasma volume replacement fluids. In itself it continues to be the subject of a great deal of research. While its role in volume replacement has been questionable, we await further research before either condemning or promoting its clinical application.

3.2.8. References

1. Peters TJ. Metabolism: albumin in the body. In: All about albumin. Biochemistry, genetics, and medical applications San Diego: Academic Press; 1996: 188-250.

2. De Feo P, Gaisano MG, Haymond MW. Differential effects of insulin deficiency on albumin and fibrinogen synthesis in humans. Journal of Clinical Investigation 1991; 88: 833-40.

3. Hutson SM, Stinson-Fisher C, Shiman R, Jefferson LS. Regulation of albumin synthesis by hormones and amino acids in primary cultures of rat hepatocytes. American Journal of Physiology 1987; 252: E291-8.

4. Johnson TR, Rudin SD, Blossey BK, Ilan J. Newly synthesised RNA: simultaneous measurement in intact cells of transcription rates and RNA stability of insulin-like growth-factor 1, actin, and albumin in growth hormone-stimulated hepatocytes. Proceedings of the National Academy of Science USA 1991; 88: 5287-91.

5. De Feo P, Horber FF, Haymond MW. Meal stimulation of albumin synthesis: a significant contributor to whole body protein synthesis in humans. American Journal of Physiology 1992; 263: E794-9.

6. Doweiko JP, Nompleggi DJ. Role of albumin in human physiology and pathophysiology. Journal of Parenteral and Enteral Nutrition 1991; 15: 207-11.

7. Yedgar S, Carew TE, Pittman RC, Beltz WF, Steinberg D. Tissue sites of catabolism of albumin in rabbits. American Journal of Physiology 1983; 244: E101-7.

8. Cochrane Injuries Group Albumin Reviewers. Human albumin administration in critically ill patients: a systematic review of randomised controlled trials. BMJ 1998; 317: 235-40.

9. Fleck A, Hawker F, Wallace PI, Raines G, Trotter J, Ledingham IM, Calman KC. Increased vascular permeability: a major cause of hypoalbuminaemia in disease and injury. The Lancet 1985; i: 781-4.

10. Sun X, Iles M, Weissman C. Physiological variables and fluid resuscitation in the postoperative intensive care unit patient. Critical Care Medicine 1993; 21: 555-61.

11. Hoye RC, Bennett SH, Geelhoed GW, Gorschboth C. Fluid volume and albumin kinetics occurring with major surgery. Journal of the American Medical Association 1972; 222: 1255-61.

12. Mouridsen HT. Turnover of human serum albumin before and after operations. Clinical Science 1967; 33: 345-54.

13. Fleck A, Raines G, Hawker F, Ledingham IM. Synthesis of albumin by patients in septic shock (abstract). Archives of Emergency Medicine 1984; 1: 177

14. Howard G, Downward G, Bowie D. Human serum albumin induced hypotension in the postoperative phase of cardiac surgery. Anaesth Intensive Care 2001; 29: 591-4.

15. Matejtschuk P, Dash CH, Gascoigne EW. Production of human albumin solution: a continually developing colloid. British J Anaesth 2000; 85: 887-95.

16. Moldave K. Eukaryotic Protein Synthesis. Annual Reviews in Biochemistry 1985; 54: 1109-1149.

■ Further Reading

Nicholson JP, Wolmarans M, Park GR. The role of albumin in critical illness. Br J Anaesth 2000; 85: 599-610.

Boldt J. The good, the bad and the ugly: should we completely banish human albumin from our intensive care units? Anesth Analg 2000; 91: 887-95.

3.3. Synthetic colloids (Dextran, gelatin, hydroxyethylstarch)

3.3.1. Introduction

Hypovolemia due to absolute or relative blood volume deficits is a characteristic feature of hospitalized patients, especially those undergoing major surgery and the critically ill. Prolonged hypovolemia leads to shock, a condition characterised by failure of the circulatory system, resulting in inadequate perfusion of tissues and organs, increased postoperative morbidity, length of hospital stay, and possibly death. Thus, an adequate restoration of intravascular volume is of paramount importance.

There has been debate since the 1960s regarding the ideal choice of fluid therapy and an extensive search is in progress to determine which solution is most suitable for the replacement of intravascular volume deficits (1-3). Parallel to the general crystalloid-colloid debate the optimal colloid for plasma volume expansion in different clinical situations is also a matter of considerable controversy. The ideal fluid should not only promptly restore the intravascular volume in order to maintain systemic hemodynamics, but should also guarantee or even improve organ perfusion and microcirculation without being associated with side effects (4) (Table 3.5).

General
• Distributed to intravascular compartment only
• Readily available
• Long shelf life
• Inexpensive
• No special storage or infusion requirements
• No special limitations on volume that can be infused
Physical Properties
• Iso-oncotic with plasma
• Isotonic
• Low viscosity
• Contamination easy to detect
Pharmacokinetic Properties
• Half-life should be 6 to 12 hours
• Should be metabolised or excreted & not stored in the body
Non-Toxic & No Adverse Effect on Body Systems
• No interference with organ function even with repeated administration
• Non-pyrogenic, non-allergic & non-antigenic
• No interference with hemostasis or coagulation
• No effect on immune function including resistance to infection
• Not causing acid-base disorders

Table 3.5: The properties of an ideal colloid.

Although the ideal fluid has yet to be found, a variety of colloid solutions are currently available for intravascular volume replacement therapy (Table 3.6). In the present chapter the pharmacological characteristics and clinical effects of currently available synthetic colloid solutions are reviewed.

Natural colloids
• Albumin 5 % - 20 % - 25 %
Synthetic colloids
• Hydroxyethyl starch
- Concentration: 3 % - 6 % - 10 %
- Molecular weight (D): 70,000 – 130,000 – 200,000 – 450,000
- Molar substitution ratio (MS): 0.4 – 0.5 – 0.62 – 0.7
• Gelatin
- Cross-linked, urea linked, succinylated
- Concentration: 3.5 – 4.0 – 5.5
• Dextran
- Concentration: 6 % - 10 %
- Molecular weight (D): 40,000 – 70,000

Table 3.6: Colloids available for plasma volume expansion.

3.3.2. Pharmacokinetik and Pharmacodynamic aspects

Total body water in the adult usually ranges from 60-70 % of body weight and is contained in two distinguishable volumes of distribution the intracellular and extracellular compartment. Fluid fluxes between the intra- and extravascular water compartments are mainly influenced by hydrostatic and colloid osmotic gradients as predicted by the Starling transcapillary fluid equilibration equation. Under physiological conditions, a near-equilibrium situation exists between forces tending to shift fluid out of the capillaries (mean capillary hydrostatic pressure, interstitial fluid colloid osmotic pressure) and one major force tending to move fluid back into the capillary bed, resulting in a net fluid flow from the capillaries to the interstitium and back to the blood circulation via the lymphatic system (Figure 3.3).

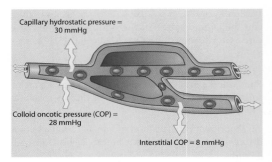

Capillary hydrostatic pressure = 30 mmHg

Colloid oncotic pressure (COP) = 28 mmHg

Interstitial COP = 8 mmHg

Figure 3.3: Hydrostatic and oncotic forces influencing the intravascular and extravascular fluid compartments.

The colloid osmotic pressure (COP) of the plasma proteins is the main factor for the retention of intravascular volume and the prevention of interstitial tissue edema. Therefore, natural and synthetic colloids are important in capillary fluid dynamics because they are the only constituents which are effective in exerting an osmotic force across the wall of the capillaries.

Colloids are large molecular weight (nominally MW > 30,000) substances that are either monodispersed, like albumin, if the molecular size and weight are uniform throughout the product; or polydispersed, if there is a variety of different molecule sizes and shapes. Pharmacological characterization of synthetic colloids includes concentration, mean molecular weight, and degree and position of substitution, as occurs with starches. The available colloid preparations differ with regard to volume-supporting capacity, intravascular half-life, their influence on hemorheological variables, and their side effect profile (4).

The initial volume effect of a colloid solution is primarily dependent on the concentration of its colloid-osmotically active molecules, while the duration of the volume effect depends mainly on the in vivo molecular weight of the solution, the configuration of the molecules, and the renal elimination characteristics for a substance (Figure 3.4).

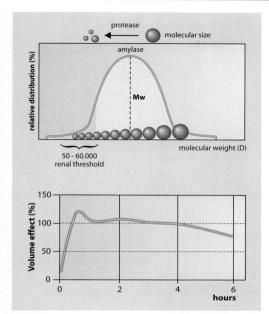

Figure 3.4: Molecular weight (D) distribution and plasma volume expanding effect of polydispersed synthetic colloids.

The COP of a colloid is the major factor influencing the initial plasma volume-expanding capacity. Intravenous infusion of a colloid with a COP equal to that of plasma will result in isovolemic effects, whereas colloid solutions with a higher COP than plasma will additionally increase intravascular volume due to resorption of interstitial fluid. Volume effects are mainly dependent on the number of molecules. Lower molecular weight particles are rapidly renally excreted in contrast to larger particles. Large molecules, in turn, only contribute minimally to the volume expansion effects; they affect viscosity and persist in the circulation.

The duration of volume stabilizing effect is also important to consider since reversibility could be important in case of fluid overload with pulmonary edema; conversely, a sustained plasma expansion seems to be mandatory to obtain prolonged hemodynamic stability in critically ill patients. It was therefore thought that a long acting colloid should be generally preferred. Unfortunately, these long acting colloids accumulate within tissues (skin, kidneys, mononuclear phagocytic system) and this may be associated with adverse effects ranging from persistent itching after repeated administration of hydroxyethylstarch solutions to

more serious consequences such as renal dysfunction and failure or impaired blood coagulation after dextran infusions (5). Other theoretical hazards and side-effects of synthetic colloid solutions will be discussed below.

3.3.3. Gelatins

Gelatins are polydispersed polypeptides produced by degradation of bovine collagen. Gelatin solutions were first used as colloids in the treatment of hypovolemic shock as early as 1915. The early solutions had a high molecular weight, which had the advantage of a significant oncotic effect but the disadvantages of a high viscosity and a tendency to gel and solidify if stored at low temperatures. Reducing the molecular weight reduced the tendency to gel but smaller molecular weight molecules could not exert a significant oncotic effect.

Three types of modified gelatin products are now available: cross-linked or oxypolygelatins (e.g. Gelifundol®), urea-crosslinked (e.g. Haemacel®), and succinylated or modified fluid gelatins (e.g. Gelofusine®) (Table 3.7).

	Urea-cross-linked gelatin	Cross-linked gelatin	Succiny-lated gelatin
Concentration (%)	3.5	5.5	4.0
Mean molecular weight (Dalton)	35,000	30,000	30,000
Volume effect (hours)	1-3	1-3	1-3
Volume efficacy (%)	80	80	80
Theoretical osmolarity (mosmol/l)	301	296	274

Table 3.7: Characteristics of the different gelatin solutions.

Although gelatins are products of bovine origin, they are sterile, pyrogen free, contain no preservatives and have a recommended shelf-life of 3 years when stored at temperatures less than 30° C. The molecular weight ranges from 5,000 to 50,000 Dalton with a mean molecular weight of 30-35,000

Dalton. The various gelatin solutions have comparable volume effects. The volume effect is less than the infused volume of gelatin, due to a rapid, but transient passage of gelatins in the interstitial space. Moreover, gelatins are rapidly cleared from the bloodstream by glomerular filtration and, to a lesser extent, undergo cleavage by proteases into small peptides in the reticuloendothelial system. Therefore, repeated infusions of gelatin are necessary to maintain adequate blood volume. This disadvantage is balanced by the fact that there are no dose limitations with gelatins, as occurs with dextran and hydroxyethylstarch.

Gelatins do not accumulate in the body and appear to be without adverse on kidney function. Although for a long time gelatins were considered not to influence blood coagulation other than by dilution, there is now increasing evidence that gelatins do influence platelet function and blood coagulation. In a recent study comparing the effects of progressive hemodilution with gelatin, saline, hydroxyethylstarch and albumin on blood coagulation, significant changes in the thromboelastogram were found after the infusion of gelatin solutions (6). The clinical relevance of the impairment of hemostasis after gelatin infusion, however, is uncertain.

All colloids used for volume therapy, including the natural colloid albumin, have the potential to induce anaphylactic or anaphylactoid reactions. The overall incidence of allergic reactions with gelatins is higher than that seen with hydroxyethylstarch, and almost comparable to that seen with dextrans (5).

3.3.4. Dextrans

Dextran is a mixture of glucose polymers of various sizes and molecular weights derived from Leuconostoc mesenteroides, bacteria isolated originally from contaminated sugar beets (Figure 3.5).

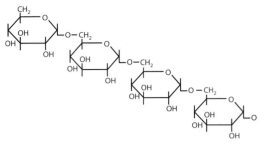

Figure 3.5: Molecular structure of dextran.

The formulations currently available are 10 % Dextran 40 (Rheomacrodex®) and 6 % Dextran 70 (Macrodex®) (Table 3.8).

	6 % Dextran 70	10 % Dextran 40
Mean molecular weight (Dalton)	70,000	40,000
Volume effect (hours)	5	3-4
Volume efficacy (%)	100	175 - (200)
Maximum daily dose (g/kg)	1.5	1.5

Table 3.8: Characteristics of different dextran solutions.

Dextrans have a dual clinical purpose and are used as plasma expanders as well as to prevent thromboembolism (7).

The colloid oncotic power of the dextran solutions is very high, due to a high water-binding capacity. One gram of dextran 40 retains 30 mL of water and one gram dextran 70 about 20-25 mL of water. Following intravenous administration dextran is almost exclusively eliminated by the kidneys. Only a small fraction transiently enters the interstitial space or is eliminated via the gastrointestinal tract. The length of time that dextran stays in the intravascular compartment is based on particle size. Approximately 60 % to 70 % of dextran 40 is cleared within 5 hours. Dextran 70 has a duration of action of 6 to 8 hours.

■ Rheologic effects

Dextran solutions were widely used to maintain circulatory dynamics during various types of shock and in the setting of ischemia-reperfusion injury. They were also used to improve blood rheologic properties, especially for decreasing blood viscosity, which should ultimately translate into improvements of blood flow in the microcirculation and then tissue perfusion. The rheologic effect of dextran 40 is especially pronounced since these solutions reduce whole blood viscosity more for the same degree of hemodilution than any other plasma substitute (8). Moreover, dextran tends to reduce harmful interactions between activated leukocytes and the microvascular endothelium ("leukocyte sticking"). These interactions play an important role in ischemia-reperfusion injury, since activated leukocytes release intermediates which are known to damage the endothelial cell membrane. Experimental studies using intravital microscopy have shown a significant reduction in this type of leukocyte-endothelium interaction at very low doses of dextran. Despite these positive macro- and microhemodynamic effects, the use of dextrans is declining in most countries because of their significant side effects.

■ Anaphylactic/anaphylactoid reactions

The dextrans cause more severe anaphylactic reactions than gelatins or the starches (5). The reactions are due to dextran reactive antibodies which trigger the release of vasoactive mediators. The incidence of these reactions can be reduced by pretreatment with a hapten. Injection of 20 mL of dextran 1000 (Promit®) a few minutes before any kind of dextran infusion should be mandatory and significantly reduces severe allergic reactions.

■ Renal function

Impaired renal function may be another problem with the use of dextran solutions (9,10). Renal dysfunction and acute renal failure after dextran infusion have been reported in patients who share several risk factors, such as preexisting renal disease, low urine output prior to dextran administration, hemodynamic instability, advanced age in combination with dehydration, or treatment with high doses of dextran for several days. Since there is no chemical toxicity of dextrans, the most likely mechanism for dextran-induced renal dysfunction may be swelling and vacuolization of tubular cells and tubular obstruction due to the production of a hyperviscous urine. It should be mentioned, however, that all hyperoncotic colloids (albumin 20 % or 25 %, hydroxyethly starch 10 %) can induce this type of renal dysfunction (9,10).

■ Hemostatic abnormalities

Dextrans have a well-documented negative effect on blood coagulation, resulting in an increased bleeding tendency (6). Dextran infusion induces a dose-dependent acquired "von Willebrand's syndrome", with decreased levels of von Willebrand factor (vWF) and associated factor VIII (VIII:c) coagulant activity. The fall in vWF and factor VIII:c after dextran administration is larger than can be explained by its dilutional effects. Besides this, dextrans also enhance fibrinolysis. These effects are greater with high molecular weight dextrans. It is therefore not surprising that in several clinical studies the administration of high doses of dextran (>1.5g dextran/kg body weight) has been associated with increased postoperative blood loss and higher transfusion requirements. Consequently, there is a maximal dosage recommendation of 1.5g dextran/kg body weight/day (about 1,500 mL for initial fluid resuscitation in an adult) to avoid serious bleeding complications.

3.3.5. Hydroxyethyl Starches

Hydroxyethyl starch (HES) refers to a class of synthetic colloid solutions that are modified natural polysaccharides. HES is derived from amylopectin, a highly branched starch which is obtained from maize or potatoes. Polymerised D-glucose units are joined primarily by 1-4 linkages with occasional 1-6 branching linkages. The degree of branching is approximately 1:20, which means that there is one 1-6 branch for every 20 glucose monomer units. Natural starches cannot be used as plasma substitutes because they are insoluble in water and rapidly hydrolyzed by circulating amylase. Substituting hydroxyethyl for hydroxyl groups results in highly increased solubility and slows hydrolysis of the compound by amylase, thereby delaying its breakdown and elimination from the blood. The hydroxyethyl groups are introduced mainly at carbon position C_2, C_3, and C_6 of the anhydroglucose residues (Figure 3.6).

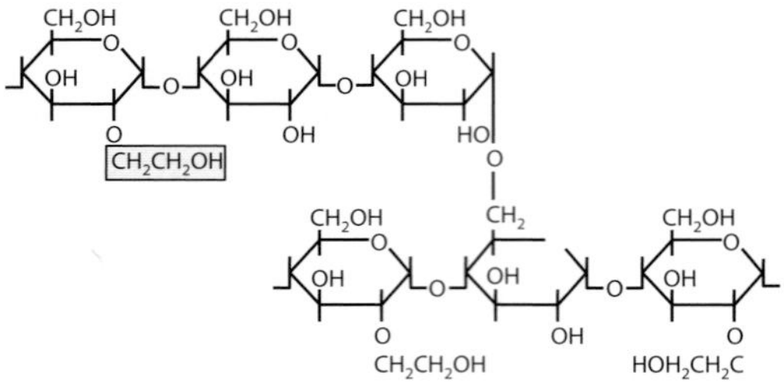

Figure 3.6: Molecular structure of hydroxyethyl starch. A segment of hydroxyethyl starch with a hydroxyethyl group is indicated.

Unlike the dextrans, which are mainly characterized by their concentration and the mean molecular weight, the pharmacokinetics of HES preparations are further characterized by the pattern of hydroxyethylation, in particular by the molar substitution and by the degree of substitution. The *molar substitution (MS) ratio* is computed by counting the total number of hydroxyethyl groups present and dividing the number by the number of glucose molecules. Currently available HES solutions have a MS of 0.4 to 0.7. For example Voluven®, a newly designed third-generation medium molecular weight HES with a molar substitution of 0.4 has four hydroxyethyl groups for every ten glucose units. The *degree of substitution (DS)* is determined by measuring the number of substituted glucose molecules and dividing this number by the total number of glucose molecules present. Another key factor in the pharmacokinetic behaviour of HES solutions, however, appears to be the C_2/C_6 *hydroxyethylation ratio*, which is possibly responsible for some side effects such as tissue accu-

mulation and bleeding complications (4). In Europe, numerous types of HES preparations with different combinations of concentration, mean molecular weight (MW), and hydroxyethylation patterns are available (Table 3.9).

It is important to distinguish between the different HES preparations, because the extent and duration of plasma volume expansion, as well as their effects on blood rheology, the coagulation system, and other clinical variables differs with respect to the specific physicochemical properties of a HES preparation (4). The water-binding capacity of HES ranges between 20 and 30 mL/g. Therefore, HES solutions have a good volume stabilizing effect. Following the infusion of HES there is initially a rapid amylase-dependent breakdown with renal excretion of up to 50 % of the administered dose within 24 hours. The hydroxyethyl residues, especially when bound to the C_2 carbon position of glucose, inhibit plasma amylase activity, hence increasing the intravascular half-life of the HES solution. A higher molecular weight and a more extensive molar substitution result in slower elimination. Smaller HES molecules (<50-60,000 Dalton) are eliminated rapidly by glomerular filtration. Renal elimination by filtration continues as larger HES molecules are hydrolysed to smaller molecules. A small amount of the administered dose is shifted into the interstitial space for later redistribution and elimination. Another fraction is taken up by the reticuloendothelial system where the starch is slowly broken down. Thus, trace amounts of the preparations can be detected for several weeks after administration.

	HES 70/0.5	HES 130/0.4	HES 200/0.5	HES 200/0.5	HES 200/0.62	HES 450/0.7
Concentration (%)	6	6	6	10	6	6
Volume efficacy (%)	70-90	100	100	130	100	100
Volume effect (hours)	1-2	2-3	3-4	3-4	5-6	5-6
Mean molecular weight (Dalton)	70,000	130,000	200,000	200,000	200,000	450,000
Molar substitution	0.5	0.4	0.5	0.5	0.62	0.7
C2/C6 ratio	4:1	9:1	6:1	6:1	9:1	4.6:1

Table 3.9: Characteristics of different HES solutions.

■ Microcirculatory effects of HES solutions

Hypovolemia may initiate a complex patho-physiologic process (e.g. stimulation of the sympathoadrenergic and renin-angiotensin systems) that may result in an inadequate tissue perfusion and decreased tissue oxygen supply. Therefore, fluid therapy should not only stabilize macrohemodynamics, but also have beneficial effects on microcirculation and tissue oxygenation. HES preparations have been successfully used for both, the treatment of intravascular volume deficits and the improvement of microcirculatory blood flow. The rheologic effectiveness of different HES preparations is determined by their high hemodilutional capacity in combination with their inherent specific pharmacological effects on red cell aggregation, platelet function, plasma viscosity, and blood corpuscle-endothelial cell interactions. In addition, vascular resistance is reduced by lowered whole blood viscosity, which will enhance venous return and increase cardiac output. The net result would be improved blood fluidity, which might beneficially influence tissue perfusion and oxygenation after HES infusion. Indeed, intravascular volume replacement with the third-generation medium molecular weight HES 130/0.4 improved tissue oxygenation in patients undergoing major abdominal surgery (11) (Figure 3.7). In contrast, equivalent volumes of a crystalloid solution (lactated Ringer's solution) were associated with a marked decrease of tissue oxygen tensions. In this study a flexible polarographic microprobe was inserted into the deltoid muscle for measurement of skeletal muscle partial pressure of oxygen. Increased tissue oxygen tension may have a clinical impact in terms of improved wound healing and less infectious complications, which has been shown in another clinical trial in patients undergoing major colon surgery. Other authors suggested that HES may be able to ameliorate capillary leakage secondary to inflammation. However, whether HES solutions are able to "seal the leak" in patients with systemic inflammatory response syndrome or sepsis, as proposed by these results, must be clarified by additional studies.

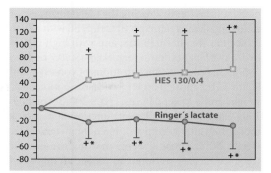

Figure 3.7: Relative changes (in %) in tissue oxygenation in patients undergoing abdominal surgery following administration of HES 130/0.4.
Differences (in percentage from baseline) of tissue oxygen tension in the two volume groups (HES with a molecular weight of 130,000 D and a molar substitution of 0.4 versus lactated Ringer's solution).

■ HES and the coagulation system

One major concern with the use of HES solutions is a possible alteration in the coagulation system (6). Imbalances in the normal hemostatic mechanisms are commonly seen in surgical patients, because of blood loss, hypothermia or activation of inflammatory processes with a subsequent imbalance of pro- and anticoagulatory pathways. Moreover, during blood loss normovolemic volume replacement with synthetic colloids inevitably leads to dilution of red blood cells, platelets, and coagulation factors. It is therefore understandable that blood coagulation becomes progressively compromised as well. The type of fluid used may also affect coagulation. Coagulation changes occur after the use of HES, but different HES preparations can have different effects on hemostasis. Several studies on impaired hemostasis with increased bleeding tendency after the use of HES have been published. The effects of HES on blood coagulation strongly depend on its molecular weight and rate of elimination and the majority of these studies used the first-generation high-molecular weight HES (hetastarch; HES 450/0.7) with a high MS (6). However, there is only very little information on the mechanism by which HES affects blood coagulation or platelet function beyond that observed after hemodilution alone. It is hypothesised that large HES molecules induce a specific decrease of von vWF and factor VIII:c by precipitation, leading to a lengthened activated partial thromboplastin time. HES has also been suggested to reduce platelet function by coating the platelet surface or inducing platelet damage. In fact, HES with a high molecular weight, high MS, and with high C2/C6 hydroxyethylation ratio (e.g. HES 450/0.7 or HES 200/0.62) reduced concentrations of von vWF and factor VIII:c more than HES with lower molecular weight and a lower MS (e.g. HES 200/0.5 or HES 130/0.4). Abnormal platelet function also occurs more often after administration of high-molecular weight HES. Thus, it seems that high-molecular weight HES preparations can induce an increased bleeding tendency, whereas HES with lower molecular weight and a lower MS are probably safe in this respect. Reliable conclusions regarding the effects of a specific HES on blood coagulation and operative bleeding will require a prospective, well-controlled, and large-scale study.

■ Interaction with renal function

Impaired renal function is one of the problems with the use of synthetic colloids and there is evidence that patients treated with HES solutions may suffer from renal dysfunction (12,13). Several hypotheses and risk factors have been proposed to explain the mechanism of renal dysfunction associated with HES administration (Figure 3.8).

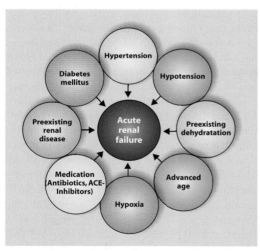

Figure 3.8: Risk factors for developing renal dysfunction.

Some histological studies have shown reversible swelling of renal tubular cells after the administration of certain HES preparations, most likely related to reabsorption of macromolecules. Swelling of tubular cells causes tubular obstruction and

medullary ischemia, two important risk factors for the development of acute renal failure. In a retrospective study, Legendre et al. reported an 80 % rate of "osmotic nephrosis-like lesions" (vacuolization of the proximal tubular cells) in transplanted kidneys after routine administration of a HES with a medium molecular weight, high MS, and high C2/C6 hydroxyethylation ratio (HES 200/0.62) to brain-dead donors (13). The lesions, however, had no negative influence on graft function or serum creatinine three and six month after transplantation. Similar tubular lesions have been described with other colloids (dextran, gelatin). The most likely mechanism of causing renal dysfunction is the induction of hyperviscosity of the urine by infusion of hyperoncotic colloids in dehydrated patients. Glomerular filtration of hyperoncotic molecules from colloids causes a hyperviscous urine and stasis of tubular flow, resulting in obstruction of the tubular lumen. Considering this pathogenesis, it can be hypothesized that all hyperoncotic colloid solutions can induce renal impairment. In the case of HES, the risk of high plasma COP and thus the risk of acute renal failure are probably increased by high concentrations of the colloid (10 % HES) or repeated administration of HES with a high in vivo molecular weight. With adequate hydration, however, using sufficient amounts of crystalloids, HES has little if any adverse effects on renal function (4). Furthermore HES solutions with a low or medium molecular weight, such as HES 130/0.4 or HES 200/0.5, did not increase the risk for renal dysfunction even when used in large amounts perioperatively.

3.3.6. Key points

- The importance of an adequate circulating volume in patients undergoing surgery as well as in the critically ill is well established. The primary goal for volume replacement therapy is to augment intravascular volume and to maintain stable hemodynamics. Microcirculatory blood flow and organ perfusion should also be guaranteed.

- There are three classes of synthetic colloid; gelatins, dextrans, and hydroxyethyl starches; each is available in several formulations with different properties which affect their initial plasma expanding effects, retention in the circulation and side-effects.

- Three different gelatin preparations are currently available, which contain a high proportion of low molecular components that are poorly retained in the intravascular space. Therefore, their volume expansion efficacy is limited and repeated infusions of gelatins are necessary to maintain an adequate blood volume. This disadvantage is balanced by the fact that there are no dose limitations with gelatins, as occurs with dextran and hydroxyethylstarch.

- Dextrans appear to be excellent plasma volume expanders and provide an improved blood rheology. Despite these positive circulatory effects, the use of dextrans is declining in most countries because of their significant side effects (allergic reactions, impaired blood coagulation and renal function). There is a maximal dosage recommendation of 1.5 g dextran/kg body weight/day

- In Europe, numerous types of HES preparations with different combinations of concentration, weight-averaged mean molecular weight, and hydroxyethylation patterns. Hydroxyethyl starches are the synthetic colloids with the pharmacological properties that are closest to natural colloids. HES preparations have been successfully used for both the treatment of intravascular volume deficits and to improve microcirculatory blood flow. Side-effects on blood coagulation and kidney function were mainly seen with first-generation high-molecular weight substances with a high degree of substitution. These side-effects are limited when modern HES preparations with a lower molar substitution and a large medium size molecule fraction are used.

3.3.7. References

1. Schierhout G, Roberts I. Fluid resuscitation with colloids or crystalloids in critically ill patients: a systematic review of randomised trials. BMJ 1998; 316:961–4

2. Choi P, Yip G, Quinonez L, Cook D. Crystalloids versus colloids in fluid resuscitation: a systematic review. Crit Care Med 1999; 27:200–10

3. Astiz ME, Rackow EC. Crystalloid-colloid controversy revisited. Crit Care Med 1999; 27:34–5

4. Boldt J. Volume replacement in the surgical patient – does the type of solution make a difference? Br J Anaesth 2000; 84:783-793

5. Laxenaire MC, Charpentier C, Feldman L. Anaphylactoid reactions to colloid plasma substitutes: frequency, risk factors, mechanisms. Ann Fr Anesth Reanim 1994; 13:301-10

6. De Jonge E, Levi M. Effect of different plasma substitutes on blood coagulation: a comparative review. Crit Care Med 2001; 29:1261-7

7. Daniel WJ, Mohamed SD, Metheson NA. Treatment of mesenteric embolism with dextran 40. Lancet 1966; 1:567–9

8. Menger M. Influence of isovolemic hemodilution with dextran and HAES on the PMN-endothelium interaction in postischemic skeletal muscle. Eur Surg Res 1989; 21:74

9. Baron JF. Adverse effects of colloids on renal function. In: Vincent JL, eds. Yearbook of intensive care and emergency medicine 2000. Berlin: Springer; 2000: 486-93

10. Moran M, Kapsner C. Acute renal failure associated with elevated plasma oncotic pressure. N Engl J Med 1987; 317:150-3

11. Lang K, Boldt J, Suttner S, Haisch G. Colloids versus crystalloids and tissue oxygen tension in patients undergoing major abdominal surgery. Anesth Analg 2001; 93:405-9

12. Cittanova ML, LeBlanc I, Legendre C, Mouquet C, Riou B, Coriat P. Effects of hydroxyethyl starch in brain-dead kidney donors on renal function in kidney-transplant recipients. Lancet 1996; 348:1620-22

13. Legendre C, Thervet E, Page B, et al. Hydroxyethyl starch and osmotic nephrosis like lesions in kidney transplantation. Lancet 1993; 342:248-9

3.4. Artificial oxygen cariers

Artificial oxygen (O_2) carriers aim at improving O_2 delivery. Artificial O_2 carriers thus may be used as an alternative to allogeneic blood transfusions or to improve tissue oxygenation and function of organs with marginal O_2 supply (1,2,3). Modified hemoglobin solutions and perfluorocarbon emulsions are currently in clinical testing. Current knowledge of artificial O_2 carriers is based on the published data of approximately 500-1000 patients dosed with these compounds and a similar number of control patients. Unfortunately, there is still a significant amount of non-published data which renders the overall assessment difficult.

The concept of augmented acute normovolemic hemodilution (augmented ANH™) will also be discussed. In augmented ANH, the patients are hemodiluted prior to surgery. During the course of the intervention, a further reduction of the hemoglobin concentration is expected. In order to maintain the oxygenation of tissues, an artificial O_2 carrier is administered. The autologous blood harvested during preoperative hemodilution is finally re-transfused at the end of surgery. Thereby, the need for allogeneic blood transfusion is reduced.

Artificial O_2 carriers can be divided into two principal groups: modified hemoglobin (Hb) solutions and emulsions of perfluorocarbon (PFC). The hemoglobin may originate from outdated human blood, be of bovine origin or genetically engineered (1,2,4). The molecule of native human hemoglobin must be modified in order to decrease O_2 affinity and to prevent rapid dissociation of the native a_2-$ß_2$ tetramer into a-ß dimers. This has been reviewed in detail previously (1,2,4).

The characteristics of O_2 transport of modified Hb solutions and PFC emulsions are fundamentally different. The majority of Hb solutions exhibit a sigmoidal O_2 dissociation curve, similar to blood (figure 3.9). The emulsions of PFC are on the other hand characterized by a linear relationship between O_2 partial pressure and O_2 content. Thus, the majority of the solutions of Hb have O_2 transport and unloading capacities similar to those of blood (figure 3.9). This indicates that even for a relatively low O_2 partial pressure, a substantial quantity of oxygen is transported, contrary to the use of the PFC emulsions, which require a relatively high O_2 partial pressure to optimize the transport of oxygen.

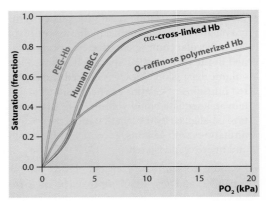

Figure 3.9: O_2 dissociation curve of native human blood (Human RBCs) and different modified Hb solutions (PEG-Hb, a-a cross-linked Hb and O-raffinose polymerized Hb) (modified according to Stowell at al. (4)).

3.4.1. Hemoglobin solutions

Efficacy of Hb solutions to transport and release O_2 in tissues has been shown in a variety of studies on animal models, including extreme hemodilution, hemorrhage, surgical trauma and sepsis (3). It has been demonstrated that treatment with a-a-Diaspirin cross linked Hb improved wound healing, stimulates proliferation of hepatic cells and decreases splanchnic bacterial translocation, in comparison with transfusion of fresh autologous blood. In septic O_2 supply dependent rats, the administration of a-a-Diaspirin cross linked Hb increased O_2 uptake similarly as transfusion of fresh

Product	Type of surgery	Number of subjects	Autologous blood harvesting	Reference	Manufacturer
O-raffinose cross-linked human hemoglobin *Hemolink™*	CABG	299	IAD	(10,13)	Hemosol Inc. http://www.hemosol.com
Bovine derived hemoglobin based oxygen carrier HBOC-201 *Hemopure®*	Major orthopedic surgery	693	None	(11)	Biopure Corp. http://www.biopure.com
	Cardiac surgery	98	None	(12)	
Perflubron emulsion *Oxygent™*	Major cancer surgery	492	ANH	(19)	Alliance Pharmaceutical Corp. http://www.allp.com

Table 3.10: Efficacy data of published phase III trials of currently developed artificial oxygen carriers. CABG = Coronary artery bypass graft surgery, IAD = Intraoperative blood donation, ANH = Acute normovolemic hemodilution.

(< 6 days old) red blood cells whereas animals treated by stored red blood cells presented a high mortality. Furthermore, a-a-Diaspirin cross linked Hb enabled extreme, virtually red blood cell free, hemodilution in pigs with absence of subendocardial ischemia at a hematocrit of 1 %. In a similar model but with a critical coronary stenosis, pigs resuscitated with a-a-Diaspirin cross linked Hb survived experimental hemorrhagic shock more frequently than animals resuscitated with albumin.

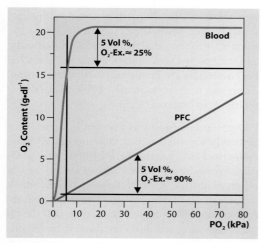

Figure 3.10: O_2 dissociation curve of native human blood (Blood) (modified according to Looker at al. (20)) and perflubron emulsion (PFC) (modified according to Keipert et al. (16)). 5 Vol % of O_2 can be offloaded by blood and by perflubron emulsion. With perflubron emulsion, however, higher arterial PO_2 values are required. Perflubron emulsion transported O_2 is more completely off-loaded than blood transported O_2 resulting in approximate O_2 extraction (O_2-Ex.) ratios of 90 % and 25 %. PO_2 denotes O_2 partial pressure.

Therefore, modified Hb solutions improved transport of O_2 and tissue oxygenation. Moreover, by the fact that they do not require cross-matching, these solutions promise to present an interesting alternative to allogeneic blood transfusions and as O_2 therapeutics, which might be of great importance also in the pre-hospital resuscitation of trauma victims or for specific conditions in intensive care medicine.

Due to genetic or chemical modifications of the native Hb molecules, the degradation of the α_2-β_2 tetramer into α-β dimers is prevented and nephrotoxicity is no longer a complication of this

solutions (5). On the other hand, all these solutions induce an increase in the systemic and pulmonary artery pressure by vasoconstriction. The mechanisms involved include nitric oxide (NO) scavenging, endothelin release and a sensitization of peripheral adrenergic receptors (1,2,4). NO produced by the endothelial cells is intended to react with the Fe^{2+} in the guanylate cyclase located in the smooth muscle cells of the vessel wall to modulate the vascular tone towards vasodilatation. It has been speculated that unpolymerized Hb molecules in particular may penetrate into the subendothelial layers of vessel walls to scavenge NO and thus induce vasoconstriction. The pressor response of hemoglobin solutions may be minimized by general anesthesia. Nevertheless, distinct vasoconstriction is viewed as a limitation in the development of hemoglobin based O_2 carriers (6) since any increase in blood pressure may aggravate blood loss in trauma victims and compromise survival. Indeed, a study in trauma victims has been prematurely terminated due to an increased mortality in patients treated with a-a-Diaspirin cross linked Hb (7), and the development of this Hb solution has been stopped after these events (8).

Still, allogeneic blood transfusions may be reduced with the use of a-a-Diaspirin cross linked Hb in patients undergoing cardiac surgery (8). In a prospective randomized multicenter study, 209 patients were allocated to receive either packed allogeneic red blood cells or up to 750 mL of a 10 % a-a-Diaspirin cross linked Hb solution when reaching a defined transfusion trigger following cardiopulmonary bypass. In the a-a-Diaspirin cross linked Hb group, 59 % of patients avoided allogeneic blood transfusions until the first postoperative day, while, by study protocol, 100 % of patients randomized to the control group had been transfused. At hospital discharge, 19 % of patients in the a-a-Diaspirin cross linked Hb group still avoided any allogeneic transfusion as compared to none in the control group. Also in emergency surgery the amount of allogeneic blood transfusions was reduced by the use of an Hb solution (9).

Three recent phase III trials in cardiac and orthopedic surgery deserve mentioning (10-12). O-raffinose cross-linked human hemoglobin in conjunction with intraoperative hemodilution reduced the need for allogeneic blood transfusions in 299 patients undergoing coronary artery bypass surgery (10). Reported side effects included a 10 % elevation of arterial blood pressure, a higher incidence of episodes of hypertension and a transient elevation of bilirubin linked to the hemoglobin metabolism (13). In the second study regarding cardiac surgery (12) 98 patients were randomized at the first postoperative transfusion decision, between a treated group receiving HBOC-201, a bovine derived hemoglobin based oxygen carrier, and a control group receiving allogeneic red blood cells transfusions. 24 % of the patients of the treated group avoided any transfusion vs. 0 % in the group controls (p < 0.05). In 693 patients undergoing major orthopedic surgery, HBOC-201 increased the percentage of patients avoiding any allogeneic blood transfusion from 0 % (patients were randomized at the first perioperative transfusion decision) to 59 % for the entire study period of 6 weeks (11). In this preliminary report (abstract) the analysis of adverse and serious adverse events were not reported (11), rendering safety assessment difficult at present time. However, the side effect profile of HBOC-201 was published recently (14). In this study, escalating doses of 0.6-2.5 g/kg doses of HBOC-201 (corresponding to infusion volumes of 380 ± 87 to 1384 ± 309 mL) were given to 42 patients and data were compared to 26 control patients receiving lactated Ringer's solution. Blood pressure was slightly but significantly higher in HBOC-201 dosed patients, a trend (p = 0.06-0.08) towards elevated postoperative lipase levels and a late methemoglobinemia (peaks at the thirst postoperative day) were observed, and in 23 of 42 patients (58 %) IgG-antiHBOC-201 antibody were detected at follow-up. In contrast, renal function, platelet count, blood coagulation parameters and general clinical laboratory values were similar in both groups (14).

Since Hb solutions are coloured, they may interfere with certain colorimetric laboratory methods currently used in clinical chemistry. In contrast, ABO and Rh typing and cross-match testing do not seem to be affected (referenced in (3)).

3.4.2. PFC emulsions

PFCs are carbon-fluorine compounds characterized by a high gas dissolving capacity (O_2, CO_2 and other gases), low viscosity, and chemical and biologic inertness (15). PFCs are virtually not miscible with water and thus need to be emulsified. A stable 60 % perflubron emulsion (58 % perfluorooctyl bromide and 2 % perfluorodecyl bromide) has been developed, which is, in general, clinically well tolerated (15).

After intravenous administration, the perflubron emulsion is being taken up by the reticuloendothelial system (RES). This uptake determines intravascular half life ($T_{1/2}$), which also depends on the total dose given. Thus, after a 1.8 g/kg perflubron emulsion dose, $T_{1/2}$ is approximately 10 hours. After the initial uptake of the PFC emulsion into the RES, the droplets of the emulsion are slowly broken down, the PFC molecules are being taken up in the blood again (bound to blood lipids) and transported to the lungs, where the unaltered PFC molecules are finally excreted via exhalation. At present time, metabolism of PFC molecules is unknown in humans (1,15).

Perflubron emulsion was assessed in a variety of hemodilution studies in animal models. At a hematocrit of 10 % a massive rise in mixed venous O_2 partial pressure and mixed venous saturation was observed in dogs. When perflubron is administred, the percentage of metabolized O_2 originating from endogenous Hb decreased, indicating that the O_2 transported by perflubron emulsion is preferentially metabolized, most likely due to its excellent O_2 unloading characteristics (16). Perflubron emulsion also improved survival of severely hemodiluted dogs undergoing cardiopulmonary bypass. In addition, after hemodilution to a Hb of 7 g/dl, mixed-venous O_2 partial pressure was higher in perflubron emulsion treated animals than in control animals. Cardiac function was also improved after perflubron emulsion administration at a Hb level of 3 g/dl. This may be explained by an increase in O_2 delivery on the level of very narrow capillaries, where the size of the particles of perflubron emulsion (~ 0.16 µm in diameter) allows their passage much more easily than for the relatively large erythrocytes (7-8 µm in diameter). Thus, the local oxygenation of tissues, and in particular of the myocardium, is increased (referenced in (3)).

Perflubron emulsion has also been used in humans (referenced in (3)). In a prospective randomized multicenter study, patients undergoing orthopedic surgery were hemodiluted preoperatively to a Hb of 9 g/dl (17). After the patients had reached a predefined transfusion trigger, they were randomized into 4 groups: A, standard of care (retransfusion of 450 ml of autologous blood at an unchanged FiO_2 of 0.4), B and C, perflubron emulsion (0.9 or 1.8 g/kg) with colloid to a total 450 ml and ventilation with an FiO_2 of 1.0 and D, infusion of 450 ml of colloid with ventilation with an FiO_2 of 1.0. Perflubron emulsion (1.8 g/kg) was most successful in reversing transfusion triggers in 97 % of patients as compared to 60 % in the control group. In addition, transfusion trigger reversal lasted longer in the perflubron emulsion 1.8 g/kg group (80 min) than in the control (55 min) and colloid groups (30 min) (17). Thus, physiological transfusion triggers may be treated at least as successful with perflubron emulsion as with autologous blood. This illustrates the remarkable capacity of perflubron emulsion to deliver available O_2 to the areas of the body which have the greatest need for it.

Also PFC emulsions have side effects. Volunteers experienced mild flu-like symptoms with myalgia and light fever and an approximately 15 % decrease in platelet count 3 days post-dosing; returning to normal by day 7 (15). However, traditional coagulation tests, bleeding time and platelet aggregation, were unaffected by perflubron emulsion. Finally, enrolment in a phase III study in cardiac surgery was voluntarily suspended in 2001 due to an apparent imbalance in adverse neurological outcome (4). Experts, however, agree that these events were not directly related to the PFC emulsion used but to the rapid blood harvesting procedure early on cardiopulmonary bypass. In fact, in the same study it was observed in a subset of patients monitored with gastric tonometry that in PFC treated patients, the gastric mucosal pH were higher, indicating an improved splanchnic oxygenation, resulting in earlier postoperative bowel movement (18).

Augmented ANH with perflubron emulsion has been shown to reduce the need for allogeneic blood transfusion in 492 patients undergoing major non-cardiac surgery. PFC-treated patients first underwent ANH to a hemoglobin of 8.0 ± 0.5 g/dl, followed by dosing with perflubron emulsion. The PFC group had significantly fewer transfusions of allogeneic and predonated autologous blood and the percentage of subjects completely avoiding transfusions was significantly higher (19). The efficacy was particularly high in patients with major blood loss (> 20 mL/kg) but already in patients with mo-derated blood loss (> 10 mL/kg) a significant reduction on allogeneic blood transfusion was observed which was sustained until hospital discharge. Although more serious adverse events were observed in the group of patients undergoing augmented ANH with perflubron emulsion, no organ system was specifically involved and overall tolerance was good (19). Again, lower platelet counts were found postoperatively in patients dosed with perflubron emulsion but this was of limited clinical relevance since neither platelet transfusion were more frequent in these patients, nor postoperative bleeding events nor postoperative allogeneic blood transfusions. In fact overall allogeneic blood products (red blood cells, fresh frozen plasma, platelets) were transfused less in the group of patients treated by augmented ANH and perflubron emulsion (19). Augmented ANH with perflubron emulsion thus appears to be a promising treatment option for patients undergoing non-cardiac surgery, in which the blood loss is moderate to high.

3.4.3. Future uses of artificial O_2 carriers

Future use of Hb solutions and PFC emulsions may include a combination of acute normovolemic hemodilution (ANH) with application of an artificial O_2 carrier during the operation, a procedure termed augmented ANH (figure 3.11). Augmented ANH is a concept in which patients will undergo ANH to relatively low hematocrit levels prior to surgical blood loss. ANH thus may be performed preoperatively or initially during the operation, but prior to the phase of major blood loss. In the phase of major surgical blood loss colloids and crystalloids will be administered to avoid hypovolemia and artificial O_2 carriers will be co-administered to maintain tissue oxygenation. As a consequence, lower hematocrit levels can be safely tolerated. Towards the end of the operation, the autologous blood harvested during ANH will be retransfused. This will increase postoperative hematocrit levels and O_2 delivery will again be provided by endogenous red blood cells. Therefore, greatly elevated arterial PO_2 values are not necessary in the postoperative period and the relatively short half life of all artificial O_2 carriers (< 24 h) will not compromise their success in reducing perioperative allogeneic blood transfusion requirement.

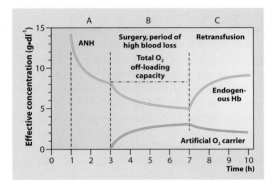

Figure 3.11A-C: Augmented-ANH (A-ANH): The concept of Augmented-ANH is split into three periods. **(A)** ANH with conventional volume replacement without the use of artificial O$_2$ carriers prior to major blood loss targeting relatively low hematocrit levels. **(B)** During surgery, when the hematocrit is expected to fall further an artificial O$_2$ carrier is given to enhance tissue oxygenation. Note, that total O$_2$ off-loading capacity from combined red blood cell based and artificial O$_2$ carrier based O$_2$ transport is maintained above the individual transfusion trigger. **(C)** Once surgical hemostasis has been achieved the ANH blood is being retransfused to increase the endogenous Hb above the individual transfusion trigger. Therefore, the decreasing contribution of artificial O$_2$ carrier based O$_2$ transport will not adversely affect oxygenation of the organism.

3.4.4. Outlook

Great progress in the development of artificial O$_2$ carriers have been achieved in recent years but no artificial O$_2$ carrier has achieved a market approval yet in the US, Canada or Europe. Achieving market approval obviously is the next major goal. A Biologic License Application has indeed been submitted in July 2002 to the U.S. Food and Drug Administration (FDA) for HBOC-201 to achieve regulatory approval. However, we should already be thinking of the necessary education of healthcare professionals. They need to understand these new concepts, the physiology and the specifics of each of these compounds. Only in the hands of the experienced can artificial O$_2$ carriers be used to benefit the patients.

3.4.5. References

1. Spahn DR, Pasch T. Physiological properties of blood substitutes. News Physiol Sci 2001;16:38-41.

2. Winslow RM. Blood substitutes. Advanced Drug Delivery Reviews 2000;40:131-42.

3. Spahn DR, Kocian R. Place of Artificial Oxygen Carriers in Reducing Al-logeneic Blood Transfusions and Augmenting Tissue Oxygenation. Can J Anaesth 2002:(in press).

4. Stowell CP, Levin J, Spiess BD, Winslow RM. Progress in the development of RBC substitutes. Transfusion 2001;41:287-99.

5. Viele MK, Weiskopf RB, Fisher D. Recombinant human hemoglobin does not affect renal function in humans: analysis of safety and pharmacokinetics. Anesthesiology 1997;86:848-58.

6. Winslow RM. alphaalpha-crosslinked hemoglobin: was failure predicted by preclinical testing? Vox Sang 2000;79:1-20.

7. Sloan EP, Koenigsberg M, Gens D et al. Diaspirin cross-linked hemoglobin (DCLHb) in the treatment of severe traumatic hemorrhagic shock: a randomized controlled efficacy trial. JAMA 1999;282:1857-64.

8. Lamy ML, Daily EK, Brichant J-F et al. Randomized trial of Diaspirin cross-linked hemoglobin solution as an alternative to blood transfusion after cardiac surgery. Anesthesiology 2000;92:646-56.

9. Gould SA, Moore EE, Hoyt DB et al. The first randomized trial of human polymerized hemoglobin as a blood substitute in acute trauma and emergent surgery. Journal of the American College of Surgeons 1998;187:113-20.

10. Carmichael FJ, Biro GP, Cheng DC. Phase III clinical trial of hemolink in conjunction with intraoperative autologous donation (IAD) in cardiac surgical patients. Artificial Cells, Blood Substitutes and Immobilization Biotechnology 2001;29:102.

11. Jahr JS. A novel blood substitute: Use of HBOC-201 (Hemopure) to decrease need for RBC: Results of pivotal trial in orthopedic surgery patients. Crit Care Med 2001;29 (Suppl.):A168.

12. Levy JH, Goodnough LT, Greilich PE et al. Polymerized bovine hemoglobin solution as a replacement for allogeneic red blood cell transfusion after cardiac surgery: results of a randomized, double-blind trial. J Thorac Cardiovasc Surg 2002;124:35-42.

13. Cheng DC, Martineau R, MacAdams C et al. Safety of Hemolink as an oxygen therapeutic in patients undergoing coronary artery bypass graft surgery. Anesth Analg 2001;92 (Suppl.):SCA3.

14. Sprung J, Kindscher JD, Wahr JA et al. The use of bovine hemoglobin glutamer-250 (Hemopure) in suergical patients: Results of a multicenter, randomized single-blind study. Anesth Analg 2002;94:799-808.

15. Riess JG. Oxygen carriers ("blood substitutes")—raison d'etre, chemistry, and some physiology. Chem Rev 2001;101:2797-920.

16. Keipert PE, Faithfull NS, Bradley JD et al. Oxygen delivery augmentation by low-dose perfluorochemical emulsion during profound normovolemic hemodilution. Adv Exp Med Biol 1994;345:197-204.

17. Spahn DR, van Bremt R, Theilmeier G et al. Perflubron emulsion delays blood transfusion in orthopedic surgery. Anesthesiology 1999;91:1195-208.

18. Frumento RJ, Mongero LM, Naka Y, Bennett Guerrero E. Preserved gastric tonometric variables in cardiac surgical patients administered intravenous perflubron emulsion. Anesth Analg 2002;94:809-14.

19. Spahn DR, Waschke K, Standl T et al. Use of perflubron emulsion to decrease allogeneic blood transfusion in high-blood loss non-cardiac surgery: results of a European phase 3 study. Anesthesiology 2003:(in press).

Volume replacement in specific clinical situations

4. Volume replacement in specific clinical situations

4.1. Volume replacement in children

Children are not little adults. This is particularly true for water and electrolyte balance. The clinically most significant changes during volume replacement occur in preterm babies, neonates, and infants. However, toddlers are also at risk of volume overload when the nature and size of the intravenous fluid volume they are administered are more than their little bodies can handle. The case report that follows is a particularly tragic example.

Case Report

M., a 3-year-old girl weighing 18 kg, was scheduled for adenoidectomy. Along with the brief anesthesia required for this procedure, the girl was given 250 mL of 5 % dextrose and electrolytes. On the ward, she received another 500 mL of 5 % dextrose until 6:00 PM. At that time the girl experienced postoperative bleeding, which the otolaryngologist considered significant enough to warrant surgical control in the OR, involving another infusion of 250 mL of 5 % dextrose. The girl received another 500 mL of 5 % dextrose overnight. On the next morning, she experienced a convulsion. On examination, she had dilated, fixed pupils. Soon afterward the patient experienced brain stem incarceration. She died from cerebral edema.

Unfortunately, this is not an isolated case. Court appointed experts in pediatric anesthesiology malpractice proceedings have, over the past two decades, reported at least 10 cases of serious postoperative neurologic damage or death due to inadequate perioperative intravenous fluid therapy in Germany alone. It is therefore imperative to become familiar with essential considerations that are unique to pediatric fluid and electrolyte management.

4.1.1. Physiology

■ Water Content

The water content of a premature baby is 95 percent that of a term neonate is 80 percent, and this decreases steadily in infants and toddlers to reach approximately 60 percent in a typical adult. Until puberty, there is no clinical need to differentiate between boys and girls in this regard. Obese children have a lower water content relative to total body weight than do lean children.

■ Distribution of Body Water

Assuming that ontogeny is a brief recap of phylogeny, the high percentage of the extracellular space in preterm infants means that the cells of premature babies are, as it were, still bathed in the environment they originally came from: the sea. The large extracellular space in preterm infants (ECS/ICS = 50 %/40 %) decreases to 40 percent in term neonates (ECS/ICS = 40 %/40 %), decreasing further to 20 %/40 % by 12 months of age, the ratio also typically found in adults (see Figure 4.1).

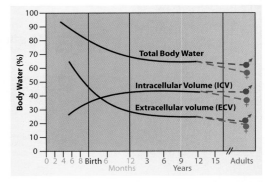

Figure 4.1: Distribution of body water as a function of age (from (9)).

This large extracellular space is clinically significant because, in relation to body weight, hydrophilic drugs need to be administered in higher doses in infants than in adults. Classical examples include suxamethonium (succinylcholine) in anesthesiology and aminoglycosides in intensive care.

The intravascular volume is 5 percent and constant across all age groups.

■ Water Turnover

Water turnover is linked to energy production and insensible water losses from the skin and respiratory tract. The differences in water turnover between infants and adults are enormous: an infant's basal metabolic rate is geared to growth, a baby weighing 3000 grams at birth will double his weight to 6000 grams within sixth months, and weigh 10 kg by his first birthday.

To achieve this feat, a neonate needs 6 to 7 mL of oxygen/kg/min - twice the oxygen demand of an adult. This large amount of oxygen is required to meet a neonate's or infant's energy requirements of 100 to 120 kcal/kg/day. Oxidation of 100 kcal equivalent of fuel produces approximately 12 mL of metabolic water per kg. Oxidation processes alone thus provide a newborn with 36 mL of water. An adult produces approximately 7 mL of metabolic water per kg of body weight, compared with as much as 12 mL per kg in an infant.

A child's growth-oriented increased basal metabolic rate results not only in substantially increased oxygen consumption but also in the production of more carbon dioxide. Expiration of this increased carbon dioxide requires increased alveolar ventilation (120 mL/kg/min in neonates compared with 50 mL/kg/min in adults).

Newborns and infants use a respiratory rate that is adapted to the gas exchange typical of neonates and minimizes breathing work at the same time. However, at 30 to 40 breaths per minute, the respiratory rate typical of this age group results in significantly greater water loss than in adults.

The water loss from the skin is larger in neonates and infants than in adults because of the greater body surface area in relation to body weight. At "neutral" temperature, the increased water loss from the skin in very premature infants (say, born in week 26 and weighing 800 grams) is initially 2.7 mL/kg/hr. Once skin keratinization is complete - this process takes about three weeks in preterm infants - water loss from the skin decreases to approximately 0.67 mL/kg/hr. Transdermal water loss in adults is as low as 0.18 mL/kg/hr. This means that very premature infants may lose up to 10 times more water through the skin than adults. In mature neonates, transepidermal water loss is still 5-fold greater (relative to body weight) than in adults (4). Also, water loss from the skin is significantly affected by numerous other factors including body temperature, ambient temperature, and phototherapy.

The daily water turnover of neonates and infants is approximately 100 mL/kg of body weight. This is equivalent to approximately 10 percent of their body weight and implies that 40 percent of their extracellular fluid is exchanged each day. Daily water intake in a 70-kg adult, on the other hand, is approximately 2000 mL, or 1/35th his body weight or 17 percent of his extracellular fluid volume. If an

adult was to follow the water turnover pattern of an infant, his water intake would be 12 to 15 liters per day (9).

■ Water Loss

Water loss occurs to:

- 10 % via the feces
- 30 to 40 % from the skin, mucous membranes, and respiratory tract
- 50 to 60 % via the urine

The kidneys start working as early as week 12 of pregnancy, and the glomeruli are fully developed by week 34/35. Fetal urine production may reach an unbelievable 1 to 2 liters per day. However, birth causes urine production to fall off sharply, probably because the mother's milk may take a few days to "come in". The newborn, therefore, must avoid volume losses as far as possible in this situation. This also means that kidney function is massively reduced in the first three days of life. This is why the glomerular filtration rate in the first three days of life is half the GFR in a 4-day-old neonate or infant. Urine output in the latter may be as much as 2 to 3 mL/kg/hr.

However, the kidneys of newborns and infants are not yet capable of concentrating the urine to the same extent as in adults. Urinary osmolarity in newborns ranges from 300 to 400 [mosmol/L]. An as-yet inadequate tubular receptor response to the release of aldosterone and antidiuretic hormone (ADH) causes substantial sodium loss. This situation has been termed "sodium loss kidney" or "physiological renal insufficiency".

In fact, the kidneys are not fully functional until after the end of the first year of life (4).

■ Cardiovascular System

Cardiac output is determined by:

- heart rate
- myocardial contractility
- intravascular volume

The cardiovascular system of children is unique in that their cardiac output, at a constant intravascular volume, is controlled almost solely by the heart rate. A child's heart is incapable of increasing its myocardial contractility, or, at best, has very limited inotropic adaptability. The heart rate of preterm infants ranges from 120 to 180 beats per minute, and that of (term) neonates ranges from 100 to 140 bpm (see Table 4.1).

	Heart Rate (bpm)	Systolic Blood Pressure (mm Hg)	Diastolic Blood Pressure (mm Hg)
Neonates	125	75 to 85	40 to 50
1 to 12 Mos	120	85	60
1 to 3 Yrs	110	90	60
3 to 5 Yrs	100	95	62
3 to 7 Yrs	100	100	65
7 to 11 Yrs	90	115	72
11 to 16 Yrs	80	120	75

Table 4.1: Heart rate of neonates, infants, and children.

Blood pressure is not a reliable indicator of intravascular volume adequacy. Conscious pediatric patients can compensate even large volume losses by increasing the heart rate; blood pressure remains constant for a long time. In fact, blood pressure falls only when there is cardiocirculatory failure. As neonates and infants are capable of vasoconstriction, blood pressure is not a useful indicator of the presence of hypovolemia.

In the anesthetized child, these compensations mechanisms are paralyzed, and volume loss will therefore be accompanied by a reduction in blood pressure.

The intravascular volume of a term neonate is 90 mL/kg of body weight; it decreases to 80 mL/kg in the second year of life. Seemingly small volume losses of approximately, 150 mL, means a 50 percent loss of the intravascular volume in a neonate and, therefore, has enormous hemodynamic consequences.

The hemoglobin content of neonatal blood is substantially higher and the hematocrit higher than those of the blood of infants and toddlers. The newborn has adapted to the low placental oxygen supply; fetal hemoglobin has high affinity for oxygen and is very effective at binding oxygen, thus facilitating placental oxygen transfer.

After birth, fetal hemoglobin is no longer needed because of the "luxuriant" 21 % oxygen content of ambient air. Fetal hemoglobin is therefore broken down, overloading the metabolic capacity of many

a newborn's liver and leading to transient neonatal jaundice. As the production of adult hemoglobin does not reach adult levels immediately, infants may experience anemia in the third month of life (Figure 4.2), which may be more pronounced in preterm infants than in term babies. During that time, the oxygen content of the infant's blood is half the normal concentration, and this reduces the blood's oxygen transport capacity, which the infant can compensate by increasing cardiac output and oxygen extraction.

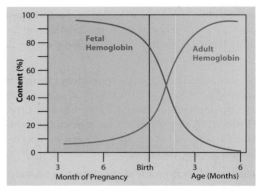

Figure 4.2: Fetal and adult hemoglobin content of a child's blood (from (9)).

4.1.2. Diagnosis and management of pediatric hypovolemia

4.1.2.1. Preliminary considerations

Intravascular volume depletion in children, like in adults, may be due to loss of:

- water and electrolytes (dehydration)
- plasma proteins
- blood

Pediatric dehydration - in neonates and infants in particular - may be a life-threatening condition. Dehydration may occur as a result of:

- diarrhea
- vomiting
- refusal to feed
- ileus
- peritonitis
- diabetes insipidus
- Addison's disease
- diuretic therapy

- salt-wasting nephropathy

Plasma loss may occur in pediatric burn patients, as it does in adult burn patients.

Blood loss occurs as a result of:

- trauma or
- intraoperative losses and spontaneous rupture of a tumor (a rare event, *e.g.*, rupture of a liver hemangioma) or a compromised organ (liver, spleen)

4.1.2.2. Diagnosis and management of disorders of water and electrolyte balances

Signs and symptoms of pediatric dehydration include:

- dry feeling or appearance inside the mouth
- hippocratic face
- poor skin turgor and tenting
- mottling of the skin as a consequence of vasoconstriction
- collapsed neck veins
- pale nasolabial triangle
- cold, clammy hands and feet (prolonged capillary refill time)
- fever (in some patients)
- decreased urinary output
- tachypnea
- tachycardia
- fall in blood pressure

In infants, the anterior fontanelle (palpable until the sutures close in the 9th to 12th months of life) is typically depressed in volume depletion.

Weight loss is a quantitative indicator of dehydration:

5 %	Mild dehydration
10 %	Moderate dehydration
15 %	Severe dehydration
>15 %	Life-threatening dehydration (volume depletion)

Because of the neonate's ability to constrict the blood vessels in the skin and muscle, blood pressure remains constant until the heart rate cannot be further increased to maintain cardiac output. Heart rate is therefore a more sensitive indicator of

hypovolemia than blood pressure. Urinary output is reduced. The core-to-peripheral temperature gradient correlates very closely with cardiac output.

Insensible perspiration is the body's way of controlling its heat balance. Perspiration is minimized in volume depletion, thus preventing heat dissipation and resulting in a rise in body temperature. The fever that develops in this situation is due to a lack of perspiration. Adequate volume replacement will reverse vasoconstriction, thus dissipating heat and lowering the fever.

Depending to a large extent on respiration, the pulse curve produced by the pulse oximeter is only a semiquantitative measure of hypovolemia. A quantitative indicator of volume depletion would be the central venous pressure, but a central venous catheter is rarely in place in children (the normal range of CVP is the same as in adults).

The laboratory provides clues as to the type of dehydration the patient has, and what components should be replaced (see Table 4.2).

Parameter	Hyponatremic (hypotonic) dehydration	Isonatremic (isotonic) dehydration	Hypernatremic (hypertonic) dehydration
Serum sodium	<130 mEq/L	130 to 150 mEq/L	>150 mEq/L
Pathogenesis	Sodium loss > water loss	Sodium loss = water loss	Sodium loss < water loss
Extracellular fluid	↓↓	↓	↓
Intracellular fluid	↑	Normal	↓
Typical disease	Addison's syndrome	Gastroenteritis	Diabetes insipidus
Frequency	10 %	70 %	20 %

Table 4.2: Types of dehydration.

Dehydration is often categorized according to serum sodium concentration:

- Isonatremic (isotonic) dehydration (serum sodium, 135 to 145 mEq/L): the lost fluid is similar in sodium concentration to the serum (*e.g.*, vomiting, diarrhea)

- Hyponatremic (hypotonic) dehydration (serum sodium, <130 mEq/L): relatively more sodium than water is lost (*e.g.*, polyuria after kidney failure)

- Hypernatremic (hypertonic) dehydration (serum sodium, >150 mEq/L): relatively less sodium than water is lost (*e.g.*, infants with fever, hyperventilation, toxicosis, diabetes mellitus)

The appropriate management of pediatric volume depletion depends on the type of dehydration (see Table 4.3):

- In isonatremic dehydration, 0.45 % sodium chloride with 5 % dextrose is usually sufficient, according to Hecker (8).

- In hypernatremic dehydration, 0.45 % sodium chloride with 5 % dextrose is indicated.

- In hyponatremic dehydration, [use the same replacement solution] as in isonatremic dehydration, adding sodium as necessary and calculated from the following formula (BW = body weight):

Sodium Needs =
(Target Na⁺ Conc (135 mEq/L)
minus
Actual Na⁺ Conc) x 0.6 x kg BW

$$\text{Sodium Needs} = (\text{Target Na}^+ \text{ Conc (135 mEq/L)} - \text{Actual Na}^+ \text{ Conc}) \times 0.6 \times \text{kg BW}$$

Daily Maintenance Fluid Requirements		
Body Weight	3 to 10 kg	100 mL of fluid per kg of BW
	10 to 20 kg	1000 mL of fluid for the first 10 kg of BW + 50 mL of fluid per kg of BW for each additional kilogram
	>20 kg	1500 mL of fluid for the first 20 kg of BW + 20 mL of fluid per kg of BW for each additional kilogram

Example:
Daily maintenance fluid requirements of a 15-kg child: 100 x 10 + 5 x 50 = 1250 mL in 24 hrs

Calculation of Additional Losses

- *Fever:* 100 mL/m² BSA per day for each degree centigrade above 37.5 °C

- *Diarrhea:* Up to 50 mL of fluid loss per kg of BW in 24 hrs

- *Vomiting:* Measure losses and replace accordingly

Table 4.3: Calculation of maintenance fluid requirements and additional losses in isotonic dehydration.

In hypernatremic dehydration, proceed as follows:

- Infuse maintenance needs plus half the fluid deficit in the first 24 hrs.

- On day 2, infuse maintenance needs plus the other half of the deficit over 24 hrs.

- In the second 24 hrs of the rehydration period, consider the use of one-third normal saline with 5 % dextrose and provide adequate potassium replacement.

It is obsolete to treat hypernatremic dehydration with 5 % dextrose, *i.e.*, free water. The rapid fall of osmolarity in the extracellular space would produce an osmotic gradient between the extracellular space and the dehydrated, hyperosmolar intracellular space. This gradient would produce a rapid influx of water into brain cells, causing cerebral edema. Serum sodium, if greater than 175 mEq/L, should therefore not be lowered by more than 10 to 15 mEq/L per day. Careful, *slow* rehydration is key to a good prognosis in hypernatremic dehydration.

Metabolic acidosis, a frequent concomitant of dehydration, is often corrected automatically by adequate volume replacement. If arterial pH is less than 7.1, administer 8.4 % sodium bicarbonate as necessary, based on the following formula:

$$8.4\text{ \% Sodium Bicarbonate (mL)} = \text{BE x 0.3 x kg BW}$$

Give half the bicarbonate dose, then repeat blood gas analysis before proceeding.

4.1.2.3. Diagnosis and management of plasma loss

Plasma loss is mainly the cause of volume depletion in burns. There are no qualitative differences in volume replacement therapy between pediatric and adult burn patients. In the acute phase, which is characterized by disrupted cell permeability of the burned skin, plasma proteins should not be replaced because of the risk of protein extravasation into burned tissue, thus worsening burn edema.

The following infusion strategy can be recommended (2).

• Using Wallace's rule of nine, estimate the total body surface area burned (TBSAB).			
• Give two-thirds normal saline with 5 % dextrose to meet maintenance needs:			
Body Weight	1 to 10 kg	100 mL per kg of BW per day
	11 to 20 kg	1000 mL for the first 10 kg of BW + 50 mL per kg of BW for each additional kilogram per day
	>20 kg	1500 mL for the first 20 kg of BW + 20 mL per kg of BW for each additional kilogram per day
Give Ringer's lactate/acetate to meet additional needs:		
Day 1	5 mL per kg of BW per %TBSAB: Infuse first half of the dose over the first 8 hrs and the second half over the next 16 hrs	
Day 2	3 mL per kg of BW per %TBSAB	
Day 3	1 mL per kg of BW per %TBSAB	

Targets of volume therapy are (2):

• Blood pressure normal for age, heart rate normal

• Urine output at least 1 mL/kg/hr (Urine output is often low despite increased CVP and adequate fluid replacement; hence the need to give furosemide at 0.5 to 2 mg/kg 4-6hrs)

• Serum electrolytes: serum sodium 138 to 145 mmol/L, serum potassium 3.5 to 4.5 mmol/L

• CVP 3 to 7 mm H_2O: higher values tend to indicate reduced excretion in the presence of excessive fluid replacement; lower values need not be corrected if the patient is in a stable hemodynamic state

• Hematocrit 30 to 40 %

• Serum osmolality 290 to 300 mosmol/kg

• Blood glucose normal

4.1.2.4. Diagnosis and management of blood loss

Intraoperative (or posttraumatic) blood loss of up to 20 percent of the estimated intravascular volume should first be replaced with an electrolyte-containing infusion fluid. Infants and toddlers are best given half normal saline with 2.5 % dextrose. The reduced dextrose concentration helps avoid hyperglycemia which often occurs when children are intraoperatively administered infusion fluids with 5 % dextrose (5). School-age children, like adults, may be given a balanced electrolyte solution.

If blood loss is greater than 20 percent of the estimated intravascular volume, children, like adults, should also receive plasma substitutes. There is no sound medical evidence to justify withholding artificial colloids from children in this situation, as has been common practice in the past.

However, studies in children are available only for the use of hydroxyethyl starch (HES). Several carefully designed and implemented studies (3,7) have found no difference between children receiving HES for volume replacement and those infused with human albumin: clinically significant differences between the two groups were observed neither in hemodynamic variables nor in laboratory parameters.

The cited research studies have, unfortunately, included only children 6 months of age and older. The use of HES in premature infants and neonates has therefore not been established. In this high-risk pediatric population it would be particularly important to know whether HES infusion interferes with blood clotting and the immune system. Interference by the latter might be due to a possible interaction with the reticuloendothelial system.

In the absence of studies of the use of synthetic colloids in preterm and newborn babies and infants up to 6 months of age, human albumin continues to be the recommended plasma expander in this age group.

The indication for blood transfusion in children varies as a function of age. A number of studies (1,6,10) of isovolemic hemodilution in pediatric patients have demonstrated that children are remarkably tolerant of low hemoglobin levels. Even at a mean hemoglobin concentration as low as 3 g/dL, children (mean age, 8.2 yrs) showed neither an increase in lactate levels as evidence of a global oxygen deficit nor hemodynamic or organ compromise (6).

To be on the safe side, a hemoglobin concentration of 6 g/dL may therefore be used as the level that indicates the need for perioperative transfusion. However, this threshold applies only to infants beyond the neonatal period. A more differentiated approach to ordering blood transfusions should be used in preterm babies and neonates (see Table 4.4).

	Hemoglobin Threshold (g/dL)
Preterm Babies	
Week 1 of Life	12
Week 2	11
Week 3	10
Week 4	9
Week 5	7
Neonates	
Days 1 & 2 of Life	13
Day 3 Through Week 2	11
Week 3	10
Week 4	9
Month 2	8
Infants Beyond Neonatal Period	
> Month 2 Through Year 1	7
Toddlers & School-Age Children	
	6

Table 4.4: Indication for blood transfusion in preterm babies and neonates as a function of age-related hemoglobin threshold (g/dL).

A differentiated approach to blood transfusion should be used regardless of whether homologous or autologous blood products are being used:

- **Whole Blood:** Nowadays rarely available from blood centers.
- **Packed Red Blood Cells (PRCs):** Buffy coat-free PRCs are of particular purity (residual white blood cell count $<1.2 \times 10^9$ WBCs per unit, platelets <5 %) and are present in additive solution (saline, adenosine, dextrose, mannitol). Buffy coat removal avoids microaggregate formation, reduces febrile transfusion reactions, and prevents buffy coat-induced acute pulmonary failure. Children, preterm babies and neonates in particular, should always receive PRCs that are as fresh as possible. Rule of thumb: give 3 mL of PRCs (or 6 mL of whole blood) per kg of body weight to raise the hemoglobin concentration by approximately 1 g/dL.
- **Irradiated Packed Red Cells:** The transmission of immunocompetent lymphocytes capable of division that may still be present in a transfused unit of PRCs may cause graft-versus-host disease (GVHD) in immunosuppressed patients. GVHD occurs only when an immunosuppressed patient is transfused with blood that contains viable immunocompetent cells such as lymphocytes. An immunocompetent body is normally capable of eliminating such transfused lymphocytes. An immunosuppressed patient, however, cannot eliminate all of those lymphocytes. The remaining immunocompetent lymphocytes recognize immuno-incompetent recipient tissues as foreign and attempt to destroy them. GVHD mainly affects the epidermis, gastrointestinal epithelium, hepatocytes, bone marrow and lymphoid tissue cells. Occurring with a latency period of 8 to 10 days, the signs and symptoms of GVHD include clinically significant erythematous eruptions, severe diarrhea (several liters per day), hepatic impairment with jaundice, transaminase elevations, *[moderate]* hepatomegaly, lymphocyte depletion of lymphoid tissues, and *[fever]*. Carrying a high fatality rate, GVHD can be prevented by irradiation of PRC units. Blood products that may contain immunocompetent cells and are to be administered to immunosuppressed patients therefore must be irradiated with 30 Gy shortly before a planned transfusion.

- **Washed Packed Red Cells:** Saline washed PRCs are prepared by blood banks, removing any residual plasma in several wash cycles as far as possible. Indications include a history of repeated severe transfusion reactions to plasma proteins (urticaria, anaphylaxis), paroxysmal nocturnal hemoglobinuria (PNH), and [prevention] of transmission of incompatible antibodies (autoimmune hemolytic anemia).

> Blood component dosage should always be individualized based on hemodynamic and laboratory parameters. The following approach can be used as a rule of thumb:
>
> - In normovolemic children, the threshold hemoglobin level for blood transfusion is 6 g/dL.
> - When transfusing packed red blood cells, complement the packed red cells with fresh frozen plasma in a ratio of 4 units of PRCs to 1 unit of FFP.
> - When a patient loses twice the blood volume, replace platelet concentrates; the threshold platelet count for a platelet transfusion is 50.000/mm³.

4.1.3. Perioperative fluid therapy in routine clinical practice

Intraoperative fluid therapy aims to meet maintenance requirements, replace fluid loss, and correct imbalances.

Maintenance needs:

- neonates until day 3 of life: 2 mL of fluid per kg of body weight per hour
- neonates from day 3 of life and infants: 4 mL of fluid per kg of body weight per hour
- infants and toddlers: 3 mL of fluid per kg of body weight per hour
- school-age children: 2 mL of fluid per kg of body weight per hour

Replacement needs are due to fluid loss via:

- evaporation from an open surgical field
- vomiting
- diarrhea
- fever

Fluid replacement needs in intraabdominal or intrathoracic surgery arise mainly from intra-operative evaporation. Replacement needs therefore must be replaced in addition to maintenance needs as follows:

- Intrathoracic surgery: 2 mL of fluid per kg of body weight per hour
- Intraabdominal surgery: 4 mL of fluid per kg of body weight per hour

Particularly careful volume replacement is necessary in preterm babies, newborns, and infants. IV fluids should always be administered by perfusion pumps in these pediatric patients. Toddlers undergoing brief surgical procedures may also be administered i.v. fluids by gravity infusion from a 250-mL bottle. Toddlers undergoing longer procedures require distinct control of fluid delivery. School-age children may be administered i.v. fluids by gravity infusion.

However, it is also essential in toddlers and school-age children to ensure that the estimated infusion volume is not grossly exceeded. A full bladder after surgery is a common cause of (seemingly) unexplained postoperative restlessness in pediatric patients.

Dextrose solutions without electrolytes for use as infusion fluids are contraindicated in pediatric patients. Infusing such solutions means infusing free water, which may lead to brain edema and possible brain tissue incarceration in the foramen magnum. Toddlers are best given half normal saline with 2.5 % dextrose. School-age children may be infused with a balanced electrolyte solution.

4.1.4. Conclusion

Volume replacement in pediatric patients, preterm babies, neonates, and infants in particular, requires an in-depth understanding and extensive experience as well as an eye for the minor losses that have such major consequences for a child's hemodynamic state.

4.1.5. References

1. Ali Hassan A, Lochbuehler H, Frey L, Messmer K. Global tissue oxygenation during normovolaemic haemodilution in young children. Paed Anaesth 1997; 7:197-204

2. Beushausen, Th. Thermische Verletzungen. In Kretz, FJ, Beushausen, Th: Das Kinder-Notfall-Intensiv-Buch, 1997; S. 451, Urban & Fischer Verlag

3. Boldt J, Krothe E, Schindler E, Hammermann H, Dapper T, Hempelmann G. Volume replacement with hy-

droxyethyl starch solution in children. Br J Anaesth 1993; 70:661-5

4. Dabbagh S, Ellis D. Regulation of fluids and electrolytes in infants and children. In Motoyama E K: Smith's Anesthesia for infants and children. 5th Edition 1990; S. 105, Th C.V. Mosby Company

5. Fösel T, Uth M, Wilhelm W, Grüneß V. Comparison of two solutions with different glucose concentrations for infusion therapy during laparotomies in infants. Infusionsther Transfusionsmed 1996; 23:80-84

6. Fontana JL, Welborn L, Mongan PD, Sturm P, Martin G, Bünger R. Oxygen consumption and cardiovascular funcion in children during profound intraoperative normovolaemic hemodilution. Anesth Analg 1995; 80:219-25

7. Hausdörfer J, Hagemann H, Heine J. Vergleich der Volumenersatzmittel Humanalabumin 5 % und Hydroxyäthylstärke 6 % (40.000/0,5) in der Kinderanästhesie. Anästh Intensivther Notfallmed 21 1986; 137-42

8. Hecker W. Dehydratationszustände im Säuglingsalter. In Kretz F J und Beushausen Th: Das Kinder-Notfall-Intensiv-Buch, Urban & Fischer Verlag 1997

9. Kretz FJ, Heidrich J. Flüssigkeits- und Volumenersatz im Säuglings- und Kleinkindesalter. In: Refresher-Course "Aktuelles Wissen für Anästhesisten". Springer Verlag 1999; S. 277

10. Perez de Sà, Békássy A, Schou H, Werner O. Bone marrow harvesting in children managed without allogenic blood. Paed Anaest. 1994; 4:375-81

4.2. Volume replacement in the elderly

4.2.1. Introduction

The world's population is getting older - at present 10 % of the population is aged 60 years or over according to a recent United Nations Report (1). It is anticipated that this trend will continue; by 2050, one in five people will be 60 years or older; and by 2150, one in three people will be 60 years or older. The fastest growing segment of the older population consists of those aged over 80. Unsurprisingly, there are dramatic differences between developed and developing countries, suggesting that improved social circumstances and healthcare in developed countries have resulted in increased longevity.

The elderly patient is usually defined as 'over 65 years old', although there is little consensus about this. Alternatively, this group may be subdivided into 'the oldest old' (over 80 years) and 'the elderly'

(aged from 65 to 80 years) (2). However, the elderly population has been described as being 'unique for its non homogeneity' (3) – the process of aging varies between individuals, some individuals will be 'good for their years' while others age prematurely.

This chapter will discuss those aspects of volume replacement of specific relevance to the elderly. The principles of volume replacement in the elderly are, broadly speaking, the same as other age groups and determined by the principles outlined in previous chapters.

Unfortunately, while the challenges of determining the appropriate therapeutic strategies are great, the evidence base is weak – most clinical trials exclude patients over 65 years. Volume replacement is most commonly used for resuscitation of the intravascular space in situations such as burns, trauma, and surgery; we will mainly discuss the surgical environment.

4.2.2. Implications of aging

There are age-related physiological changes to all organ systems, which result in a reduced functional reserve in this group. An increased incidence of many diseases in the elderly, on this background of diminished reserve, probably accounts for the relatively high mortality and morbidity observed following surgery (4,5). In considering the challenges of appropriate volume replacement in the elderly population it is appropriate to review the effects of ageing in terms of changes in physiology, pharmacology and the impact of an ever increasing incidence of morbidities.

Being older brings with it a greater risk of dying. It has been repeatedly demonstrated that age is an independent risk factor for death following for example, elective or emergency surgery. The commonest diseases associated with ageing are hypertension, renal disease, atherosclerosis, myocardial infarction, chronic lung disease, cardiac failure and diabetes mellitus.

4.2.2.1. Physiology and pathology

■ Cardiovascular system

Priebe has extensively reviewed age-related physiological and pathological changes in the cardiovascular system (6). Clinically relevant alterations in physiology include: increased myocardial and vascular stiffness, blunted β-adrenoceptor responsiveness and autonomic reflex dysfunction. Decreased left ventricular compliance, due to increased myocardial stiffness, results in higher cardiac filling pressures. For these reasons the elderly may be more sensitive to fluid overload.

Cardiovascular disease is more common in the elderly and occurs on the background of the age-related changes to the cardiac and vascular systems described. Following acute myocardial infarction, mortality and complications are increased in comparison with younger patients; there is a higher incidence of silent myocardial ischaemia. Cardiac failure is common; however systolic dysfunction should be distinguished from diastolic dysfunction - about 40 % of patients aged over 60 years with symptoms of congestive cardiac failure have preserved systolic function (6). Conduction abnormalities are more common and are poorly tolerated in the elderly. Arrhythmias may be caused or exacerbated by inappropriate volume or drug therapy causing electrolyte disturbance. Importantly, the elderly are more likely to be taking cardiac medication.

■ Respiratory system

Changes with age are both anatomical e.g. decreased chest wall compliance, decreased lung elastance, decreased ventilatory muscle strength and physiological e.g. increased work of breathing, decreased response to hypoxaemia and hypercapnia. Closing volume increases with age; by 65 years closing volume equals tidal volume in the sitting position (3). Thus, the elderly may be more susceptible to ventilation/perfusion mismatching as a result of hypovolaemia or impaired gas exchange as a result of pulmonary oedema.

There is a decrease in arterial oxygen tension (PaO_2) with age; this increases the risk of hypoxaemia, for example in the perioperative period. In turn, reduced oxygen delivery may impair end-organ perfusion, contributing to myocardial ischaemia (6).

■ Renal system, fluid and electrolytes

Renal function declines with age, and diseases affecting the kidney become more prevalent. Approximately 0.5 to 1 % of nephrons are lost with each year of life, mostly from the cortex. However the serum creatinine is generally unchanged, since skeletal muscle mass decreases at a similar rate to glomerular filtration rate (GFR) (3). The elderly mainly lose cortical nephrons; the remaining medullary nephrons have less concentrating ability and thus excrete more free water.

The elderly demonstrate impaired homeostatic mechanisms of sodium and water balance.

Renal tubular response to aldosterone is reduced, as is the ability to conserve sodium. Conversely, there is a slow response to a sodium load due to a reduced GFR and impaired tubular function (7). There is a decreased ability to excrete a free water load and mobilise third space fluid. The elderly have increased osmoreceptor sensitivity - they release more antidiuretic hormone (ADH) in response to hypertonicity; however end-organ response to ADH is altered so that water retention is less than in the young (3,7). Thirst perception is altered and associated disease states may reduce the amount of fluid ingested.

Conservation and delayed excretion of sodium and free water could potentially result in hypervolaemia or hypovolaemia in the setting of abnormal cardiovascular compensatory mechanisms (6).

Body composition changes with age; there is a relative decrease in total body water and a relative increase in body fat. In 80 year olds, there is a 10 to 15 % loss of total body water, mostly limited to the intracellular compartment; plasma volume and extracellular volumes are maintained (3). This results in altered proportions of extracellular and intracellular fluids; there is decreased intracellular fluid in proportion to total body water but a relative increase in extracellular fluid (7).

The elderly are vulnerable to electrolyte disturbances due to abnormal physiology, pathology and iatrogenic causes. Most serum electrolytes do not alter in the healthy elderly; however serum potassium may increase with age, although total body potassium is reduced (7). There is significant risk of hyponatraemia after surgery, due to ADH secretion provoked by surgical stress, chronic disease and medications such as thiazide diuretics. This may be compounded by use of hypotonic maintenance fluids after surgery. Finally, the elderly are at risk of hyper- and hypo-kalaemia due to concurrent medication, disease, or inadequate potassium supplementation in intravenous maintenance fluids.

■ Other systems

Liver mass and blood flow decreases with age such that the functional reserve of the liver becomes inadequate (3). Therefore, the hepatic processes of metabolism, biotransformation, and protein synthesis may be inadequate, especially following surgery or critical illness.

There are multiple age related changes in the central nervous system, including loss of receptors and afferent conduction pathways, slower nerve conduction and decrease in brain cell mass and cell number (3). Changes in the autonomic nervous system result in impairment of baroreceptor responsiveness, postural response and vasoconstrictor response. The effect of many drugs on the central nervous system, e.g. opioids and benzodiazepines, is increased; in addition metabolism and excretion of these drugs is affected by age-related deterioration in hepatic and renal function. The elderly are especially susceptible to confusion, compounded by change of environment when hospitalised.

Finally, loss of connective tissue and thinning of skin makes elderly patients more susceptible to the injurious effects of interstitial oedema. Degenerative joint disease results in loss of mobility, so that development of oedema has a dramatic effect in furter reducing mobility.

4.2.2.2. Pharmacology

The incidence of adverse drug reactions is greater in the elderly than in young adults. This may reflect either alterations in pharmacokinetics and pharmacodynamics with age, or polypharmacy. As fluids used for volume replacement may be considered to be 'drugs', and medication taken by the elderly may affect their fluid and electrolyte status, these changes will be briefly considered.

The relative decrease in total body water in the elderly results in a smaller volume of distribution of water-soluble drugs. Lipid soluble drugs have a larger volume of distribution, due to the relative increase in body fat. Decrease in hepatic mass results in reduced clearance of some drugs, while presystemic metabolism may be reduced. An age-related decline in renal function reduces excretion of drugs such as digoxin.

Non steroidal anti-inflammatory drugs (NSAIDs) may induce renal failure in the elderly, particularly

in conjunction with other renal insults such as hypovolaemia, sepsis, or major surgery. The high prevalence of cardiovascular disease means that many older patients take drugs such as diuretics, digoxin and ACE inhibitors, which cause electrolyte disturbance. All of these drugs therefore influence the choice of volume therapy in elderly patients.

4.2.3. Volume replacement in the elderly

4.2.3.1. General principles

The National Confidential Enquiry into Perioperative Deaths (NCEPOD) Report for 1999 entitled 'Extremes of Age' (5) stated that 'fluid management in the elderly is often poor; it should be accorded the same status as drug prescription. Multidisciplinary reviews to develop good local working practices are required.' It must be appreciated that the clinical situation determines volume replacement strategies – resuscitation differs from maintenance. Thus appropriate strategies in the operating theatre may differ from those in the intensive care unit, even in the same patient (7).

The options of fluid administration in the elderly are the same as for other age groups. Volume replacement may be achieved with colloids or crystalloids; balanced electrolyte or saline based formulations; isotonic or hypotonic solutions; and blood products or oxygen carrying solutions (e.g. stroma free haemoglobin or perflurocarbon).
The triad of "what, when and how much" is the core of decision-making in volume replacement therapy. The "what" remains highly controversial, but the "when" is less controversial as no-one seems to doubt that maintaining a well hydrated patient, particularly the elderly is in their best interest. However, the "how much" still presents us with two extreme camps: "the wet and the dry". Many people favour the generous administration of fluid to ensure maintenance of end organ perfusion, which carries a risk of iatrogenic tissue oedema; whereas others favour the avoidance of iatrogenic oedema for its perceived deleterious effects (8).
In the NCEPOD report (5), a retrospective analysis, it was noted that many elderly patients in the sample had a large fluid intake and/or poor urine output post-operatively. Although these deaths

may be interpreted as being due to fluid overload resulting in pulmonary oedema, these observations may also be explained by failure to adequately treat hypovolaemia resulting in organ dysfunction e.g. renal failure. Two randomised studies have demonstrated improved outcome, in particular hospital stay, in elderly surgical patients receiving colloid fluid challenges guided by invasive intraoperative haemodynamic monitoring (11).

Overall, sensible general principles of volume replacement in the elderly are:

- You must give enough of whatever you choose promptly and with the appropriate level of monitoring.

- You should only ever worry about giving an elderly patient too much fluid if they are inadequately monitored, in an inappropriate environment or you are the wrong person for the job. The NCEPOD report (5) highlights the importance of 'high dependency' facilities, which are frequently the appropriate environment for optimal fluid management of the elderly patient peri-operatively.

4.2.3.2. Types of volume replacement

The choice of volume replacement fluid has been discussed at length in previous chapters. We will briefly refer to some specific studies in the elderly.

The electrolyte composition of administered fluids may contribute to the development of acid-base derangement in the elderly surgical patient. In particular, administration of saline to patients results in a hyperchloraemic metabolic acidosis. A randomised trial has examined the effects of administration of a hetastarch formulated in a balanced electrolyte solution, with those of a hetastarch formulated in saline in 47 elderly patients undergoing major surgery (9). This study demonstrated hyperchloraemic metabolic acidosis and impaired indices of splanchnic perfusion, assessed by gastric tonometry, in the saline group when compared to the balanced electrolyte group. Although the trial was halted after 47 patients (original power analysis required 62 patients), due to concerns about adverse effects of the metabolic acidosis, the findings were highly statistically significant.

Kumle et al. assessed the effect of different colloids on renal function in patients undergoing major abdominal surgery (10). Elderly patients (>65 years)

and younger patients, with normal preoperative renal function, were randomised to receive 6 % low molecular weight hydroxyethyl starch, 6 % medium molecular weight hydroxyethyl starch, or modified gelatin as volume replacement, in addition to crystalloid maintenance therapy. Markers of renal function included creatinine clearance and fractional sodium clearance; these were measured intra-operatively and until the third post-operative day. The study failed to demonstrate a negative effect on renal function in patients receiving any of these colloids; predictably baseline creatinine clearance was lower in the elderly patients. The authors concluded that all of these colloids may be safely used in elderly patients without causing renal dysfunction. However the trial excluded patients known to have renal dysfunction, therefore the conclusion may not be extended to this group.

Physicians vary greatly in their choice of volume replacement fluid, although most would agree that it is appropriate to use crystalloids to meet maintenance fluid requirements. The choice of fluid for resuscitation during surgery, trauma or burns, i.e. crystalloid, colloid, or blood, is controversial. As described by Smith and Lumb (7), 'the controversy exists in the minds of practitioners, it probably does not bear continuance in patient management protocols' - many studies have compared crystalloid with colloid use, but a clinically important difference has failed to be demonstrated.

4.2.3.3. Peri-operative volume replacement

In addition to the elderly patient's diminished physiological reserve and co-morbidity, the type of surgery determines the strategy for peri-operative volume replacement. Major surgery, associated with significant blood loss and fluid shifts, increases the challenge of optimal volume replacement. Specific operations e.g. trans-urethral resection of prostate (TURP) and pneumonectomy raise specific problems in fluid and electrolyte management.

■ Pre-operative management

Elderly patients may be intravascularly deplete prior to surgery for multiple reasons including: reduced thirst, excessive pre-operative fluid restriction, inadequate maintenance intravenous fluids, diminished renal capacity to conserve sodium and water, fluid losses associated with disease, and effects of diuretics (6). Hypovolaemia is poorly tolerated and may exacerbate the hypotensive effect of induction agents, volatile anaesthetics and positive pressure ventilation. Equally, the elderly are more sensitive to fluid overload (4,6) and appropriate monitoring of volume therapy should be used to prevent this.

The dynamic response to volume therapy may be measured by measuring pressures – e.g. central venous pressure (CVP), pulmonary artery occlusion pressure (PAOP), or by measuring flow – cardiac output or stroke volume response. Increasingly, proponents of 'pre-optimisation' of high risk elderly surgical patients would advocate measurement of flow rather than pressure to guide volume replacement strategies. Boyd et al. (12) demonstrated a dramatic improvement in mortality and morbidity in high risk surgical patients (median age over 65 years in both groups), by deliberately increasing the oxygen delivery index to more than 600 mL/min/m^2 in the protocol group. This was achieved by admitting the patient to intensive care pre-operatively, inserting invasive monitoring including a pulmonary artery catheter (PAC), and using a combination of colloid, blood and dopexamine to achieve the target oxygen delivery. Although this study involved a number of interventions, it is likely that the additional fluid given to the protocol group (median 633mL preoperatively) compared to the control group (450 mL preoperatively) accounted for some of the benefit.

Although debate about the risks and benefits of pulmonary artery catheter use continues, it is reasonable to suggest that elderly surgical patients undergoing major surgery benefit from admission to critical care pre-operatively. In this environment, volume status can be optimised prior to the surgical insult.

■ Intra-operative management

Elderly surgical patients are more likely to require invasive monitoring e.g. continuous arterial and central venous pressure monitoring intraoperatively, than younger patients. Insertion of a urinary catheter to allow monitoring of hourly urine output is often necessary. Use of a pulmonary artery catheter has been advocated to guide volume replacement (7), although other methods of cardiac output and stroke volume measurement

may be used such as the oesophageal Doppler monitor (ODM).

The Cochrane database of sytematic reviews has attempted to determine the optimal method of fluid volume optimisation during surgery for hip fracture (11). Unfortunately, only two studies were assessed to be of sufficient quality to answer the review question. The first of these studies was a prospective randomised trial of use of the ODM in 40 elderly patients undergoing hip fracture repair, demonstrated faster recovery and reduced hospital stay. In the intervention group, the ODM was used to guide repeated colloid fluid challenges; this group received significantly more colloid and had a significant increase in stroke volume measured by the ODM than the control group.

In the second study, 90 elderly patients were randomised into three groups; conventional intraoperative fluid management, additional colloid fluid challenges guided by CVP, and additional colloid fluid challenges guided by ODM. In both CVP and ODM groups, patients received a greater volume of fluid, and were deemed fit for hospital discharge more quickly than the group receiving no invasive haemodynamic monitoring. The Cochrane reviewers concluded that these methods of optimisation may reduce hospital stay; however further studies are required.

Many authorities urge caution in intraoperative volume replacement, due to the perceived risk of post-operative pulmonary oedema following prolonged extracellular water expansion (4,8). Elderly patients undergoing thoracic surgery e.g. lobectomy or pneumonectomy are especially vulnerable to pulmonary oedema, although it has not been conclusively demonstrated that post-pneumonectomy pulmonary edema is related to volume of fluid administered (8). A combination of cautious monitored volume replacement and use of inotropes and vasoconstrictors is probably the best compromise in this group.

Management of volume therapy in patients undergoing prostate resection is complicated by infusion of large volumes of bladder irrigation fluids by the urologist. Regular intra-operative monitoring of serum sodium is recommended for these patients.

■ Post-operative management

Hopefully, post-operative volume therapy consists of fluid maintenance rather than resuscitation.

This may not be the case in the setting of ongoing haemorrhage or inadequate intra-operative volume therapy resulting in organ dysfunction.

Holte et al. (8) highlight the potential post-operative problems of administration of large volumes of crystalloid, and recommend future randomised studies of 'high' versus 'low' intra-operative fluid regimens.

Elderly surgical patients will frequently require admission to a critical care facility in the post-operative period.

4.2.3.4. Critical care

Volume replacement strategies for the elderly in critical care are likely to be more restrictive than those used during surgery, especially in the setting of acute lung injury. However, the principles of monitoring response to volume therapy still apply.

The benefits of early 'goal-directed' therapy in elderly patients (mean age 67 in intervention group) with severe sepsis have been demonstrated in a randomised trial by Rivers et al. (13). These benefits included reduced in-hospital mortality and reduced severity of organ dysfunction. The intervention group received treatment with crystalloid, colloid, blood and vasoactive agents according to a protocol based on measurement of central venous pressure, mean arterial pressure and central venous oxygen saturation. During the first 72 hours of treatment, there was no difference in fluid volume administered or inotrope use between intervention and control groups. However, those patients receiving 'goal-directed' therapy received greater volumes of fluid, and more frequently received blood transfusion and inotropic support in the initial 6 hours of treatment, when compared to controls. This study suggests that the timing of volume replacement is important – early intervention prevents subsequent cardiovascular collapse and organ dysfunction.

4.2.3.5. Trauma/Burns

Volume replacement strategies follow the principles already described for surgery. It is important to highlight that elderly trauma or burns patients have a significantly higher mortality than younger patients.

4.2.3.6. Blood therapy in the elderly

The 'transfusion trigger ' for red cell transfusion in the elderly must be determined on an individual basis after an assessment of risks and benefits to the individual. Blood transfusion has been discussed in another chapter; we will confine our discussion to those issues of specific relevance to the elderly.

In the elderly surgical population, perioperative anaemia is common, either due to the effects of blood loss, or due to chronic disease e.g. renal failure or malignancy (2). Increasingly, a restrictive transfusion strategy is being employed in critical care – with haemoglobin concentrations being maintained at 7-9 g/dL rather than 10-12 g/dL (14). It is uncertain whether this is applicable to the elderly population in general. Many physicians would advocate maintaining haemoglobin concentrations of 10 g/dL in patients with known or suspected ischaemic heart disease. Unfortunately, it can be difficult to diagnose ischaemic heart disease in the elderly population due to reduced physical activity (6).

A retrospective study by Wu et al (15) demonstrated a reduction in 30-day mortality in elderly patients with acute myocardial infarction with blood transfusion if the admission haematocrit was less than 33 %. However, of patients whose admission haematocrits were more than 36 %, patients receiving blood transfusion had a higher risk of death than those not transfused. Patients with lower haematocrits on admission had a higher 30-day mortality rate.

4.2.3.7. Miscellaneous including palliative care

Fluid may be administered to the elderly via the subcutaneous route. This route is used to maintain hydration in the palliative care setting, and has even been suggested for pre-operative fluid therapy (7).

4.2.4. Conclusions

The elderly provide the clinician with multiple challenges in delivering appropriate volume replacement therapy due to the non-homogeneity of the population, changes in physiology, and associated pathology. The evidence base for therapy is unfortunately small in this age group. However, available evidence supports the administration of volume therapy guided by measurement of response, such as cardiac output or stroke volume.

As the proportion of the elderly in the population continues to increase, further research is needed into volume replacement in this group in a range of clinical settings.

4.2.5. References

1. The ageing of the world's population. Population Division, Department of Economic and Social affairs, United Nations Secretariat.

Available at: http://www.un.org/esa/socdev/ageing/agewpop.htm. Accessed May 31, 2003

2. Suttner SW, Piper SN, Boldt J. The heart in the elderly critically ill patient. Curr Opin Crit Care 2002; 8: 389-394

3. Oskvig RM. Special problems in the elderly. Chest 1999; 115: 158S – 164 S

4. Jin F, Chung F. Minimizing perioperative adverse events in the elderly. Br J Anaesth 2001; 87: 608-624

5. NCEPOD. Extremes of age. The 1999 report of the National Confidential Enquiry into Peri-operative Deaths.

6. Priebe H-J. The aged cardiovascular risk patient. Br J Anaesth 2000; 85: 763-778

7. Smith HS, Lumb PD. Perioperative management of fluid and blood replacement. In: McLeskey CH, ed. *Geriatric Anesthesiology*. Williams & Wilkins, 1997; 13-28

8. Holte K, Sharrock NE, Kehlet H. Pathophysiology and clinical implications of perioperative fluid excess. Br J Anaesth 2002; 89: 622-632

9. Wilkes NJ, Woolf R, Mutch M et al. The effects of balanced versus saline-based hetastarch and crystalloid solutions on acid-base and electrolyte status and gastric mucosal perfusion in elderly surgical patients. Anesth Analg 2001; 93: 811-816

10. Kumle B, Boldt J, Piper S et al. The influence of different intravascular volume replacement regimens on renal function in the elderly. Anesth Analg 1999; 89:1124

11. Price J, Sear J, Venn R. Perioperative fluid optimization following proximal femoral fracture. Cochrane Database of Systematic Reviews; 1, 2003

12. Boyd O, Grounds RM, Bennett ED. A randomised trial of the effect of deliberate perioperative increase of oxygen delivery on mortality in high-risk surgical patients. JAMA 1993; 270: 2699-2707

13. Rivers E, Nguyen B, Havstad S et al. Early goal-directed therapy in the treatment of severe sepsis and septic shock. New Engl J Med 2001; 345: 1368-1377

14. Hebert PC, Wells G, Blajchman MA et al. A multicenter, randomised, controlled clinical trial of transfusion requirements in critical care. New Engl J Med 1999; 340: 409-417

15. Wu WC, Rathore SS, Wang Y et al. Blood transfusion in elderly patients with acute myocardial infarction. New Engl J Med 2001; 345: 1230-1236

4.3. Volume replacement strategies in trauma patients

4.3.1. Introduction

Trauma is the fourth-leading cause of death in the USA (1). Adequate volume therapy appears to be a cornerstone of managing the trauma patient. In a prospective review of 111 consecutive patients who died in hospital after admission for treatment of injuries, the most common defects in patients` management were related to inadequate fluid resuscitation (2).

> Volume deficits are often present in trauma patients and may result in the development of post-trauma multiple organ failure (MOF) on the intensive care unit (ICU) (Figure 4.3). In addition to obvious and invisible blood loss, fluid deficits may also occur secondary to generalized alterations of the endothelial barrier resulting in diffuse capillary leakage.

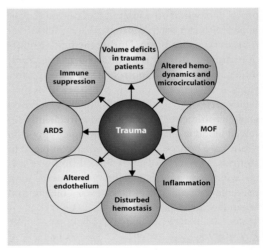

Figure 4.3: Sequelae of volume deficits in the trauma patient.

Crystalloids, human albumin (HA), hypertonic solutions, and various synthetic colloids are available to treat trauma-related volume deficits. The crystalloid/colloid dispute has been enlarged to a colloid/colloid debate because aside from the natural colloid albumin, several synthetic colloids are widely used as plasma substitutes.

In trauma patients, aggressive prehospital fluid administration ("in the field") has been common practice for more than 25 years. Some recent studies, however, have shown that early volume restoration before definite hemostasis has been performed may result in accelerated blood loss, hypothermia, and dilutional coagulopathy (3). Thus it has been recommended that volume replacement should not be started early ("permissive hypotension"; "scoop and run principle"). In the following, the controversy between delayed fluid resuscitation and early (field) volume replacement should not be intensified, but the different volume replacement strategies in the trauma patient should be reviewed. Trauma patients are different from cardiac surgery patients, patients with malignancies undergoing surgery or septic patients and thus volume replacement strategies should be separately reviewed for this kind of patients.

4.3.2. What is so specific with the trauma patient?

Trauma is often associated with blood loss. Hemorrhage-related hypovolemic shock after trauma can be divided into 3 phases:

- phase I is the period from injury to operation for control of bleeding (predefinite care)
- phase II is the period immediately during and after the operation
- phase III is the period of the trauma patient on the intensive care unit (ICU; postdefinite care)

Trauma-related hypovolemia may be associated with flow alterations which are inadequate to fulfill the nutritive role of the circulation. Many of the manifestations of organ failure after successful primary resuscitation after trauma may result from peripheral (micro-) circulatory derangements. In spite of achieving "normal" systemic hemodynamics it is not guaranteed that perfusion in all organs and tissues is maintained as well. During low output syndrome (LOS) the organism tries to compensate perfusion deficits by redistribution of flow to vital organs (e.g. heart, brain) resulting in an underperfusion of other organs (splanchnic bed, kidney). Inflammatory mediators and

vasopressors are released in this situation and are of particular importance for development of impaired perfusion.

Recent evidence suggests that the endothelium is not only a passive barrier between the circulating blood and the tissue, but may also be markedly involved in the regulation of microcirculatory blood flow by producing important regulators of the vascular tone (e.g. prostaglandins, nitric oxide, endothelins, angiotensin II). The regional regulation of blood flow is likely due to be a balance between systemic mechanisms (e.g. the autononous nervous system) and other more locally active blood flow regulators. One important approach to improve perfusion in this situation appears to be the use of adequate volume. Our pathophysiological knowledge on the importance of the endothelium in modulating microcirculation and inflammation has increased, however, the influence of different volume replacement strategies on endothelial function has to be elucidated.

Another important aspect of fluid therapy in the traumatized patient is the risk of inducing interstitial edema. Tissue edema is related to an imbalance in the sum of the Starling forces across capillary membrane or an increase in protein permeability, by which an increase in fluid flux to the interstitial space is promoted. A decrease in membrane integrity, an increase in hydrostatic pressure, and a decrease in intravascular colloid oncotic pressure (COP) will induce fluid movement across the microvascular membrane and may produce interstitial tissue fluid accumulation (e.g. pulmonary edema). Moreover, endothelial swelling may occur by which organ perfusion is further disturbed (Figure 4.4).

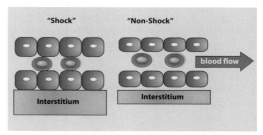

Figure 4.4: Endothelial swelling by trauma-related shock and subsequent reduction in (capillary) blood flow.

4.3.3. Volume replacement strategies in the trauma patient

The infused fluid may stay in the intravascular compartment or equilibrate with the interstitial/intracellular fluid compartments. Different mechanisms are involved in the control of volume and composition of each compartment including the antidiuretic-hormone-(ADH)-system, the renin-angiotensin-aldosteron-system (RAAS), and the sympathetic-nervous-system (SNS). The principal action of this systems is retention of water in order to restore water or intravascular volume deficits, to retain sodium in order to restore the intravascular volume, and to increase hydrostatic perfusion pressure by vasoconstriction. Enhanced activity of this systems is known to occur in stress situations, e.g. in trauma. If water or intravascular volume deficits and the stress-related stimulus of ADH, RAA and SNS are additive, volume therapy may inhibit this process through counter-regulatory mechanisms. Several attempts to attenuate the activity of ADH and RAAS by administering different amounts of crystalloid solutions were made. ADH production is dependent on the maintenance of the extracellular volume and, particularly the intravascular compartment. Administration of a restricted amount of crystalloids could replace a previous water deficit, but replacement of intravascular volume deficit would require much more volume to inhibit the activation of all these systems.

> It can be expected that replacement only of water will not inhibit the normal response of ADH and RAAS, whereas administrating a combination of crystalloids and colloids (replacement of water deficit and simultaneous guarantee of sufficient intravascular volume) may achieve this goal.

The magnitude and duration of the volume effect of a fluid will depend on the specific water binding capacity of the substance, and an how much of the infused substance stay in the intravascular space. The commonly used solutions for volume replacement differ markedly with regard to changes of COP, initial volume effects, and duration of intravascular persistance.

4.3.3.1. Allogenic blood

The risk of transmission of viral diseases has generally resulted in a more strict use of allogeneic blood. Lowering hematocrit and arterial oxygen content is not deleterious since compensating mechanisms are able to guarantee tissue oxygenation and systemic oxygen transport. When non-blood plasma substitutes are used to replace volume deficits, the margin of safety may become compromised especially in patients with significant coronary obstruction. There is an increasing risk of a discrepancy between myocardial oxygen requirements and available subendocardial oxygen supply, which may result in deterioration of myocardial performance. The "optimal" hematocrit levels, however, remains undetermined. Transfusion of allogenic blood in patients with a hemoglobin level of 8 to 10 g/dl appears to be without benefit with regard to tissue perfusion or oxygenation (4). In acute trauma, much lower hemoglobin levels are often seen and well tolerated - presumed normovolemia is present. Aside from its infectious problems, transfusion of allogenic blood may even have detrimental effects on organ perfusion, oxygenation, and immune function (5,6). In a comprehensive retrospective review of 5,366 trauma patients, blood transfusion was an independent predictor of infection, even when mechanisms of injury, injury severity score and the presence of shock were taken into consideration (6). Since allogenic blood is mostly not available in the acute trauma phase, its use is limited to patients' management in the emergency department, the operation rooms or the ICU. Blood and blood products should be restricted in this situation to treat severe anemia and coagulopathy after acute bleeding has been stopped.

4.3.3.2. Crystalloids

Hypotonic (e.g. dextrose), isotonic (e.g. saline solution), and hypertonic crystalloids (e.g. 7.5 % saline solution) have to be distinguished when using crystalloids for volume replacement. Crystalloids are freely permeable to the vascular membrane and are therefore distributed mainly in the interstitial and/or intercellular compartment. Infusion of 1,000mL of saline infusion resulted in plasma volume expansion of approximately 200mL, thus only 25 % of the infused crystalloid solution remains in the intravascular space, whereas 75 % extravasates into the interstitium. Dilution of plasma protein concentration may also be accompanied by a reduction in plasma colloid oncotic pressure (COP) subsequently leading to tissue edema. It has been shown in animal experiments that even a massive crystalloid resuscitation is less likely to achieve adequate restoration of microcirculatory blood flow compared to a colloidal-based volume replacement strategy (7). In a trauma-hemorrhagic animal model, persistent microcirculatory inhomogeneity despite normal macrohemodynamics was documented after crystalloid resuscitation (8). In an experimental trauma-hemorrhage model either colloids (dextran) or crystalloids (Ringer's acetate) were used to replace blood loss after surgical trauma (9). The crystalloid group showed significantly larger amount of tissue water in muscle and jejunum than the colloid-treated group of animals.

4.3.3.3. Colloids

4.3.3.3.1. Albumin

Albumin is a naturally occurring plasma protein. The molecular weight of albumin is approximately 69 kD. Albumin may have some additional specific effects aside from its volume replacing properties. The importance of albumin may related to its transport function for various drugs and endogenous substances, e.g. bilirubin, free fatty acids. Albumin has also been reported to possess beneficial effects on membrane permeability secondary to free radical scavenging. These effects, however, were shown only experimentally and all available clinical studies did not demonstrate any of these beneficial effects in comparison with synthetic plasma substitutes.

4.3.3.3.2. Dextran

Dextran is a glucose polymer that is available in two preparations of different molecular weights and concentrations: 6 % dextran 70 (average molecular weight 70 kD) and 10 % dextran 40 (average molecular weight 40 kD). The increase in plasma volume after infusing 1,000 mL of dextran 70 ranged from 600 to 800 mL. Some negative side-effects of dextrans have been well described including coagulation abnormalities resulting in increased bleeding tendency and severe life-treatening hypersensitivity reactions. Dextrans are

going to be replaced in several countries by other synthetic colloids because of these adverse effects.

4.3.3.3.3. Gelatins

Gelatins are modified beef collagens. Due to its low molecular weight average (approximately 35 kD), intravascular half-life of gelatin infusion is only short (approximately 2 hrs) and gelatins are supposed to be the least effective colloids. This disadvantage is balanced by the fact that there are no dose-limitation with gelatin. Gelatin is listed by the World Health Organization as an essential drug, in the USA, however, gelatin was abandoned in 1978 due to its high incidence of hypersensitivity reactions. Although the raw material is from beef, gelatins appears to be free of risk of prion transmission.

4.3.3.3.4. Hydroxyethyl starch (HES)

HES is a high polymeric glucose compound that is manufactured through hydrolysis and hydroxyethylation from the highly branched starch amylopectin. The different HES preparations are characterized by concentration (3 %; 6 %; 10 %), molar substitution (MS [0.4; 0.5; 0.62; 0.7]), and the mean molecular weight (MW [low-molecular weight [LMW]-HES: 70 kD; medium-molecular weight [MMW]-HES: from 130 to 270 kD; high-molecular weight [HMW]-HES: 450 kD]). Several different HES preparations are commercially available in Europe, whereas in the USA only the first generation HMW-HES (hetastarch; concentration: 6 %; Mw: 450 kD; MS: 0.7) is approved for volume replacement.

4.3.3.3.5. Hypertonic solutions

Enthusiasm has been expressed for hypertonic solutions (HS) or hypertonic-colloidal solutions (HHS) in the treatment of hypovolemic shock in trauma patients. The positive effects of these solutions were described in several experimental and clinical studies. HS appear to improve cardiovascular function on multiple levels - displacement of tissue fluid into the blood compartment, direct vasodilatory effects in the systemic and pulmonary circulation, reduction in venous capacitance, and positive inotropic effects through direct actions on the myocardial cells. The main mechanism of action of hypertonic solutions is rapid mobilization of endogenous fluid and subsequent plasma volume expansion. Due to the hypertonicity of the solutions, only a small volume of fluid (approximately 4mL/kg) is necessary to effectively restore cardiovascular function ("small volume resuscitation" principle). The initial improvement in cardiovascular function (e.g. increase in cardiac output) seems to be mediated by the hypertonicity of the solution, whereas the solute composition does not seem to be important. Beneficial effects of hypertonic saline solution were reported to be rather transient. Thus, hypertonic solutions were often mixed with colloids (dextran or HES), and these solutions showed significant prolongation of its efficacy (Table 4.5).

	HyperHaes ™ (Fresenius, Germany	RescueFlow™ (BioPhausia, Sweden)
Electrolyte concentration	7.2 % NaCl	7.5 % NaCl
Sodium concentration	1,232 mmol/l	1,283 mmol/l
Theoretical osmolarity	2,464 mosmol/l	2,567 mosmol/l
Colloid	hydroxyethyl starch	dextran
Colloid concentration	6 %	6 %
Mean molecular weight (kD)	200	70
Indication	severe volume deficit	severe volume deficit

Table 4.5: Characteristics of hypertonic colloidal solutions.

4.3.4. Unwanted effects of different volume replacement regimens in trauma patients

All fluids used for volume replacement in the trauma patient have merits and demerits.

4.3.4.1. Allergic reactions

Use of crystalloids is not associated with anaphylactic reactions. Severe dextran-associated anaphylactic reaction are widely known in their frequency and severity. Even prophylactic administration of monovalent hapten dextran cannot completely avoid this reaction. Gelatins are at risk to produce a larger number of anaphylactoid reactions compared with starch preparations as shown in a large trial including approximately 20,000 patients (10). Gelatins appear to be associated more often with severe, life-threatening anaphylactoid reactions, whereas this appears to be very rare after infusion of HES (10).

4.3.4.2. Influence on coagulation and increased bleeding tendency

Coagulopathy is a common complication of hemorrhagic shock. Additionally, resuscitation-associated hemodilution may alter hemostasis by lowering the concentration of clotting proteins. Use of **crystalloids** has been supposed to be without negative influence on coagulation except for that attributed to hemodilution. Recent studies have demonstrated an increased coagulability at hemodilution with saline. **Albumin** is considered to be the colloid with the least negative influence on coagulation, although procoagulatory or anticoagulatory effects (e.g. inhibiting platelet aggregation, enhancing the inhibition of factor Xa by antithrombin III) have been described with albumin. **Dextrans** are the plasma substitutes with the most widely accepted negative effects on hemostasis increasing bleeding tendency. Using dextran both VIIIR:Ag and VIIIR:RCo levels decrease significantly. With reduced VIIIR:RCo there is a reduced binding to platelet membrane receptor proteins GPIb and GPIIb/IIIa which resulted in a decreased platelet adhesion. **Gelatins** have been judged to possess no negative effect on coagulation. However, considerable negative effects on hemostasis were also demonstrated with gelatin. Changes in coagulation has most often been reported with the use of **hydroxyethylstarch** (12). However, the different HES preparations have to be distinguished concerning their influence on the hemostatic process (13). High molecular weight HES (HMW-HES, hetastarch) diminished concentrations of VIIIR:Ag and VIIIR:RCo more than HES with lower molecular weight (LMW-HES); platelet aggregation abnormalities have also been observed after infusion of HMW-HES. A substantial body of evidence supports the concept that HES with medium molecular weight (MMW-HES: 200 kD or 270 kD) and especially low MS (0.4; 0.5) have significantly less negative effects on blood clotting (68).

4.3.4.3. Tissue edema

Factors contributing to tissue edema formation are venous congestion, reduced COP, arteriolar vasodilation/venous vasoconstriction, disorganisation of interstitial matrix, increased endothelial permeability, and lymphatic dysfunction. COP appears to be an important aspect in determining fluid shift between the intravascular and interstitial compartment. Manipulation of COP appears to be promising for guaranteeing adequate intravascular volume. Controversy still exists whether the choice of fluid for restoration of circulating volume is able to limit development of tissue edema. Dilution of serum protein by massive administration of crystalloids lowers COP with the risk of progressive expansion of the interstitial space. In a non-trauma experimental peritonitis model, crystalloid infusion resulted in more pronounced endothelial cell swelling and decreased systemic capillary cross-sectional area compared with volume therapy with colloids (13).

Maintenance of COP by albumin administration has been postulated to be a desirable goal. However, in patients with impaired vascular endothelial integrity (e.g. trauma patient), albumin may pass into the interstitial compartment and fluid will subsequently shift from the intravascular to the interstitial space. A rapid and profound increase in transcapillary escape rate of radiolabelled albumin has been described within 6 hours of surgery (14). Comparing crystalloid infusion, 5 % albumin, 6 % dextran, and HES there was a greater rise in extravascular lung water (EVLW) in albumin- than in HES-treated patients. In severely ill patients it was shown that addition of albumin resulted in more signs of pulmonary failure than in patients without albumin infusion which appears to be most likely due to increased leaking into the interstitial space (15). In inflammatory-related capillary leak, HES has been reported to have 'occlusive` effects on damaged capillaries subsequently limiting extravasation of fluid (16).

4.3.4.4. Renal function

Renal dysfunction in trauma patients may develop for several reasons including unsufficiently treated hypovolemia. Crystalloids have no specific negative effects on renal system except that they may not restore blood volume adequately. The effects of the different colloidal volume replacement regimen are controversially discussed. In patients with excessive fluid deficits, glomerular filtration of hyperoncotic colloids (dextran, 10 % HES, 25 % albumin) causes a hyperviscous urine and stasis of tubular flow resulting in obstruction of tubular lumen. HES molecules and gelatin molecules are eliminated by glomerular filtration. Gelatin has almost no significant damaging effects on kidneys. In a retrospective analysis of patients undergoing kidney transplantation and in whom HES with a high MS (0.62) was infused, "osmotic-nephrosis-like lesions" were documented (17). This phenomenon, however, did not have negative effects on graft function 3 and 6 months after transplantation. In a study in intensive care patients, HES (200/0.62) resulted in significantly higher incidence of renal failure compared to a comparable group of patient who have received gelatin (18). Fortunately, the authors distinguish between different types of starches, and state that the results of the study may not be applicable to more rapidly degradable HES specifications. Use of HES 200/0.5 over 5 days in a study in trauma ICU patients was without negative effects on renal function compared to a control group in whom albumin was administered (19).

4.3.4.5. Dose limitations

Dose limitations have to be considered only when using synthetic colloids. Gelatin and dextrans are naturally occuring substances and both are fully metabolized in man. Nevertheless, a dose- limitation exists for dextrans (approximately 2,500 mL/day) most likely because higher doses are associated with severe bleeding complications. All available HES preparations are stored and may accumulate pending on the used preparation. Nevertheless, dose limitations exist for all HES preparations (ranging from 20 mL/kg to 50 mL/kg).

4.3.4.6. Immune function

Traumatic injury is known to induce intense alterations in circulatory homeostasis and cell-mediated or humoral immunity (20), subsequently trauma patients showed evidence of generalized inflammation. These sequelae of trauma predispose to the development of post-trauma sepsis or systemic inflammatory response syndrome (SIRS). The mediators of immunosuppression secondary to trauma are not definitely elucidated. Endotoxins and tissue metabolic products resulting from cellular hypoxia, shock proteins and hormonal mediators (e.g. catecholamines) are suspected to take part in this process. Polymorphonuclear cells (PMNs) are supposed to be key mediators of tissue injury and organ failure in this situation. While neutrophils are essential for bacterial killing, they paradoxically have the capacity to injure host tissue. The accumulation of activated neutrophils appears to play a key role in the pathogenesis of SIRS and development of multiple organ failure (MOF). The interactions of neutrophils with endothelial cells are regulated by complementary adhesion molecules, which are present on these cells. Soluble forms of some of adhesion molecules have been identified in the circulating blood. They appear to be excellent markers of inflammation and endothelial activation or damage. The effects of exclusive use of 10 % HES 200/0.5 or 20 % albumin for volume replacement over 5 days in severely (non-septic) traumatized ICU patients on plasma levels of circulating adhesion molecules were assessed in a prospective randomized studied (21). Plasma levels of soluble adhesion molecules were markedly higher than normal at baseline in all patients. During the study period soluble adhesion molecules did not differ between HES- and HA-treated patients indicating no negative effect of the synthetic colloid HES on endothelial function.

4.3.5. Volume replacement in trauma patients: analysis of the literature

The American College of Surgeons Classes of Acute Hemorrhage specified 4 classes of acute hemorrhage using a blood loss ranging from up to 750 mL to >2,000 mL and some additional variables (e.g. blood pressure, urine output, etc.) (22). Fluid replacement should be performed with crystalloids exclusively (3:1 rule). There is no place for infusing (synthetic) colloids in these recommendations.

4.3.5.1. Results from meta-analyses: Crystalloids and colloids

We are living in times of meta-analyses and evidence based medicine (EBM) analyses. The use of different volume replacement regimens has been examined with the help of these analyses.

- A meta-analysis from 1989 revealed a possible reduction in mortality when crystalloid solutions were used in traumatized patients (23). In this analysis, 5 trauma studies were included, two were from 1981, one from 1979, one from 1978, and one from 1977.

- The use of colloids was associated with increased incidence of death in a meta-analysis from Schierhout and Robertson from 1998 (24). Seven trauma studies were included in this meta-analysis - 3 of them used hypertonic/hyperoncotic solutions, 2 albumin, 1 dextran, and another 1 gelatin. Summerising all 37 analysed studies, resuscitation with colloids was associated with in an increased absolute risk of mortality of 4 % (or four extra death for every 100 patients resuscitated).

- In the Cochrane EBM analysis from 1998 on volume replacement, four trauma studies were included - one was from 1977, two were from 1978, and one was from 1983 (25). The message of this EBM analysis was that albumin "kills our patients" (for every 17 patients treated with albumin there was one additional death).

- One meta-analysis from 1999 distinguished between trauma patients and other kind of patients (e.g. cardiac surgery, critical care patients) (26). Four trauma studies were included, all of them were over 17 years old. All kinds of colloids were compared to crystalloid-based resuscitation. There were no differences between the two volume replacement strategies.

An objection towards all meta-analyses is that patients with different diseases had different kinds of fluids.

> The physico-chemical properties of the various synthetic colloids have mostly been neglected in all meta-analyses. Because of the important differences between individual colloids, it appears not to be appropriate to summarize all colloids in a "colloid group".

It is a main problem with most meta-analyses that they include studies >15 years old. Important innovative strategies have been developed in managing the trauma patient in the last 15 years including improved monitoring techniques, ventilation strategies, feeding, and others that also may have influence patient's disease. Finally, mortality was used as the endpoint of volume replacement in all meta-analyses. However, mortality was not the endpoint of most of the volume replacement studies and it is unclear whether mortality is helpful to find the "optimal" volume resuscitation strategy.

4.3.5.2. Volume replacement with hypertonic solutions

Treatment of trauma-related hypovolemia using hypertonic (and hyperoncotic) solutions should be assessed aside from the "classical" colloid/crystalloid or colloid/colloid debate because this represents a special issue. This strategy is mostly used only in the early (field) resuscitation of hemorraghic hypovolemia.

- In a meta-analysis of the efficacy of hypertonic 7.5 % saline/6 % dextran in trauma patients, 9 (original) studies were analysed (27). The analysis revealed no significant improvement in outcome after infusion of hypertonic saline solution, whereas use of hypertonic saline plus dextran (HSD) "may" be superior compared to isotonic volume groups.

- In a recently published meta-analysis (Cochrane Review) from 2002 comparing crystalloids with hypertonic solution, no beneficial influence of the hypertonic solutions on outcome was found (28).

In most studies on hypertonic volume replacement in trauma patients, a fixed amount of either volume was given (250 mL). It has to be doubted whether 250 mL of isotonic crystalloids given in the control patients is adequate to treat a hypovolemic trauma patient. Hemodynamics were either improved or without differences compared to the use of crystalloids. No negative influence on hemostasis, bleeding or use of packed red cells was documented.

4.3.6. Conclusions

In the severe hypovolemic trauma patient adequate volume restoration appears to be essential to stave off noncompensatory, irreversible shock (29,30). Lengthy uncorrected hypovolemia will jeopardize survival by continuous stimulation of various vasopressors and mediator cascades.

> Prolonged underresuscitation of the hypovolemic trauma patient may have fatal consequences for organ function (e.g. kidney, splanchnic perfusion, brain).

Vigorous optimization of the circulation - at least when surgical hemostasis has been achieved - is a prerequisite to avoid development of MODS in the trauma patient (Figure 4.5). This manoeuvre is aimed at guaranteeing stable macro- and micro-hemodynamics while avoiding excessive fluid accumulation in the interstitial tissue. Blood volume is restored more rapidly with colloids than with crystalloids, colloids are more efficient resuscitative fluids than crystalloids, and colloids are a more efficient regimen of guaranteeing microculatory flow than crystalloids.

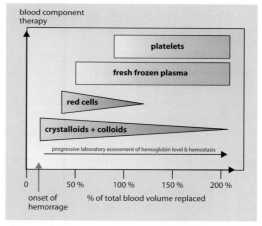

Figure 4.5: Stepwise approach of volume therapy in the trauma patient.

Only few studies are available comparing different volume replacement protocols exclusively in trauma patients. Based on these few studies, the strict recommendations published on the "best" volume replacement strategy in the hypovolemic trauma patient are surprising. It is mostly unclear from which studies these recommendations are derived from.

It is time to leave the emotional atmosphere of discussing the most appropriate volume replacement strategy in trauma patients and to concentrate on the scientific basis of this problem. When looking at the age-old "crystalloid/colloid" therapy, the only appropriate answer to the question "are you a crystalloid or colloid user?" in trauma patients is: "yes". But this doesn´t tell you the answer to the question, which is it: cristalloid/colloid?

4.3.7. References

1. MacKenzie EJ, Morris JJA, Smith GS, Fahey M. Acute hospital costs of trauma in the United States: implications for regionalized systems of care. J Trauma 1990; 30:1096-1103

2. Deane SA, Gaudry PL, Woods P, et al. The managment of injuries - a review of death in hospital. Aust NZJ Surg 1988; 58:463-469

3. Bickell WH. Are victims of injury sometimes victimised by attempts at fluid resuscitation? Ann Emerg Med 1993; 22:225-226

4. Hebert P, Wells G, Blajchman A, et al. A multicenter randomized, controlled clinical trial of transfusion requirements in critical care. N Engl J Med 1990; 340:409-417

5. Landers DF, Hill GE, Wong KC, Fox IJ. Blood transfusion- induced immunomodulation. Anesth Analg 1996; 82:187-204

6. Agarwal N, Murphy JG, Cayten CG, Stahl WM. Blood transfusion increases the risk of infection after trauma. Arch Surg 1993; 128:171-177

7. Funk W, Baldinger V. Microcirculatory perfusion during volume therapy. Anesthesiology 1995; 82:975-982

8. Hein LG, Albrecht M, Dworschalk M, Frey L, Brückner UB. Long-term observation following traumatic-hemorrhagic shock in the dog: a comparison of crystalloids versus colloidal fluids. Circ Shock 1988; 26:353-364

9. Schött U, Lindbom LO, Sjöstrand U. Hemodynamic effects of colloid concentration in experimental hemorrhage: a comparison of Ringer`s acetate, 3 % dextran-60 and 6 % dextran-70. Crit Care Med 1988; 16:346-352

10. Laxenaire M, Charpentier C, Feldman L. Reactions anaphylactoides aux subitutes colloidaux du plasma: incidence, facteurs de risque, mecanismes. Ann Fr Anest Reanimat 1994; 13:301-310

11. Warren BB, Durieux ME. Hydroxyethylstarch: safe or not? Anesth Analg 1996; 84:206-212

12. Treib J, Haass A, Pindur G. Coagulation disorders caused by hydroxyethyl starch. Thromb Haemost 1997; 78:974-983

13. Morisaki, Bloos F, Keys J, et al. Compared with crystalloid, colloid therapy slows progression of extrapulmonary tissue injury in septic sheep. J Appl Physiol 1994; 77:1507-1518

14. Fleck A, Raines G, Hawker F, et al. Increased vascular permeability: a major cause of hypalbuminaemia in disease and injury. Lancet 1995; i:781-784

15. Rackow EC, Mecher C, Astiz ME, et al. Effects of pentastarch and albumin infusion on cardiorespiratory function and coagulation in patients with severe sepsis and systemic hypoperfusion. Crit Care Med 1989; 17:394-398

16. Vincent JL. Plugging the leaks? New insights into synthetic colloids. Crit Care Med 1991; 19:316

17. Legendre C, Thervet E, Page B, et al. Hydroxyethyl starch and osmotic-nephrosis-like lesions in kidney transplantation. Lancet 1993; 342:248-249

18. Schortgen F, Lacherade JC, Bruneel F, Cattaneo I, Hemery F, Lemaire F, Brochard L. Effects of hydroxyethylstarch and gelatin on renal function in severe sepsis: a multicentre randomized study. Lancet 357:911-916

19. Boldt J, Müller M, Mentges D, Papsdorf M, Hempelmann G. Volume therapy in the critically ill: is there a difference? Intensive Care Med 1998; 24:28-36

20. Dorman T, Breslow MJ. Altered immune function after trauma and hemorrhage: what does it all mean? Crit Care Med 1994; 22:1069-1070

21. Boldt J, Müller M, Heesen M, Martin K, Hempelmann G. Influence of different volume therapies and pentoxifylline infusion circulating soluble adhesion molecules in critically ill patients. Crit Care Med 1996; 24:385-391

22. Miller RD. Update on blood transfusions and blood substitutes. Anest Analg 1999; 88 (suppl):71-78

23. Velanovich V. Crystalloid versus colloid fluid resuscitation: a meta-analysis of mortality. Surgery 1989; 105:65-71

24. Schierhout G, Roberts I. Fluid resuscitation with colloids or crystalloids in critically ill patients: a systematic review of randomised trials. BMJ 1998; 316: 961-964

25. Cochrane Injuries Group Albumin Reviewers. Human albumin administration in critically ill patients: systematic review of randomised controlled trials. BMJ 1998; 317:235-239

26. Choi P, Yip G, Quinonez L, Cook D. Crystalloids versus colloids in fluid resuscitation: A systematic review. Crit Care Med 1999; 27: 200-210

27. Wade CE, Kramer GC, Grady JJ, Fabian TC, Younes RN. Efficacy of hypertonic 7.5 % saline and 6 % dextran-70 in treating trauma: a meta-analysis of controlled clinical studies. Surgery 1997; 122:609-616

28. Bunn F, Roberts I, Tasker R, Akpa E. Hypertonic versus crystalloid fluid resuscitation in critically ill patients (Cochrane Review). The Cochrane Library, Issue 3, 2002

29. Sommers MS. Fluid resuscitation following multiple trauma. Crit Care Nurse 1990; 10:74-81

30. Henry S, Scalea TM. Resuscitation in the new millenium. Surg Clin North Am 1999; 79:1259-1267

4.4. Volume replacement in the burned patient

4.4.1. Introduction

Patients who sustain a burn injury exceeding 20-30 % of the total body surface area (TBSA) are most likely to develop a burn shock within a few hours. This is due to loss of fluid from the circulation, mainly into the interstitial space, leading to hypovolemia and hemoconcentration. There is release of a multitude of mediators, both locally and systemically, which may deleteriously affect vital organs even if circulating volume is restored. The potential mediators include free radicals, components of the complement and of the kallikrein-kinin systems, histamine, serotonin, cytokines, and arachidonic acid metabolites. The coagulation-fibrinolytic system is important both locally in the development of progressive ischemia and systemically in distant organ failure and widespread intravascular coagulation (1,2). With proper therapy shock may be avoided but the fluid given will shift to a considerable extent into the interstitial space. Increased diffusion distances may endanger tissue vitality, e.g. in partially damaged tissue, and edema can interfere with healing (3-5). The swelling of the tissues may restrict airway patency and increase the pressure within the abdomen or in muscle compartments and may necessitate surgical decompression (6,7).

According to the Two-Hit model (8), the burn injury initially cause hypovolemia and insufficient organ perfusion, along with activation of cascade systems and the release of pathogenic mediators. Hypoperfusion of the gastrointestinal tract is associated with endotoxemia or even bacteremia. The condition is usually reversible but if the metabolic situation remains sufficiently severe, or if an invasive infection develops, there may be widespread transcription of proinflammatory molecules, leading to a sepsis-like state.

Actually, the delineation of the pathophysiology of the immune system in initial burn shock to that in bacterial sepsis is unclear. Following a burns injury, there is early activation of the nuclear factor kappa B (NF-κB) (9) which seems pivotal in regulating the transcription of critical enzymes (e. g. inducible nitric oxide synthase, cyclo-oxygenase-2), increases the formation of several cytokines and promotes a sepsis-like state and organ failure (10). Several of the molecules involved in the inflammatory cascade in sepsis are indeed released early after a burn, notably IL-2, IL-6, IL-10 (11). Nevertheless, the Two-Hit paradigm remains clinically useful. Early resuscitation is rewarding to blunt the impact of subsequent complications.

Clinically, septic reactions are most often seen later after the injury and may reflect microbial invasion of the airways, growth on exposed tissue, under an eschar or in any other focus. Signs like altered mental status, tachypnea, hyperthermia or hypothermia, prolonged paralytic ileus, thrombopenia, leukocytosis or unexplained leukopenia, acidosis and hyperglycemia then herald sepsis. Procalcitonin levels are elevated after a major burn but are further increased with bacterial sepsis (12). The septic insult puts additional strain on a patient who may be vulnerable from the primary injury, with increased metabolism, impaired blood – tissue exchange and, in some cases, disturbed function of vital organs such as lungs, heart and kidneys. Failure of one or several organ systems may ensue early or late in the clinical course.

This short review will focus on the initial fluid treatment after a surface burn but preexisting disease, mechanical trauma, airway burn or inhalation of toxic compounds may complicate the clinical condition. Even though general agreement exists as to the importance of rapid treatment, there is no general consensus regarding how this should be done, appropriate goals for resuscitation, and how the procedure should be monitored. We willingly admit that this account is subjective in the sense that some procedures suggested are not well supported by outcome studies, and inference is sometimes made from observations in other fields of critical care, notably so in sepsis patients.

4.4.2. General management

Burned patients should receive oxygen by mask immediately. Similarly, an increased value of carboxyhemoglobin may indicate treatment with pure oxygen and intubation should be considered. Edema of the face and/or neck will increase over time and the airways should then be secured, particularly if the patient is to be transported to a burn center. Airway burn is an indication for intubation. This procedure, however, requires sedation and so increases the risk for circulatory instability and for respiratory infection (13).

Escharotomy and perhaps fasciotomy may be necessary before or after transport to facilitate ventilation and to save injured extremities. Burned skin releases toxic compounds (14) and is usually excised early (within 2-3 days). Extensive surgery necessitates transfusion of red cells and plasma may be indicated for specific coagulation disorders.

In burns exceeding 20 % TBSA oxygen consumption and catabolism are increased, with enhanced lipolysis and gluconeogenesis. A thermoneutral environment reduces the metabolic need (15). Enteral nutrition should be started early and may decrease the translocation of microorganisms in the gastrointestinal tract. There is a substantial evaporation from the burn wounds, which may amount to 100-200 mL/h and m^2 TBSA, depending on air humidity, the depth of the wound, and whether dressings are applied and whether the wounds are excised or not.

4.4.3. Pathophysiology

4.4.3.1. The burn wound

Thermal injury may coagulate tissue, leading to irreversible cessation of circulation. In an intermediate surrounding zone of stasis, blood flow will be present but the tissue may later be indistinguishable from the zone of coagulation. In less damaged tissue there is, following initial vasoconstriction, a zone of vasodilatation (2). In the latter, partially damaged tissues, there is also intracellular edema, due to energy shortage within the cells, affecting the sodium-potassium pump mechanism (16-18).

In less damaged tissue, there is an immediate extracellular edema that increases during the first hours. This edema has been attributed to increased capillary pressure and decreased capillary permeability towards macromolecules. However, it has long been realized that these changes are insufficient to account for the entire edema development and the formation of osmotically active molecules in the interstitial tissue has been invoked (19). Later, it was shown by Lund and coworkers (20) that there is thermal destruction of the extracellular matrix with degradation and unraveling of the collagen triple helix. A negative pressure (inhibition pressure), that may amount to minus 150 mm Hg, may result from the denaturation of the crosslinking,

creating an osmotic and hydrostatic gradient and immediately resulting in edema.

Thus, the capillary injury and the "suction" of fluid into the tissues imply that the shift of fluid into the burn wound cannot be limited by using colloidal fluids in the resuscitation (21). The time course of the normalization of the intercellular matrix in burnt skin is not well known but structural recovery and lymph drainage from the tissue must play an important role.

4.4.3.2. Generalized edema

Interstitial edema, albeit less prominent, can develop in non-injured tissues as well and this fluid volume may exceed that accumulated within directly injured tissue (22-24). There are reports that distant capillary beds have been affected even after burns of 6-8 % TBSA (25,26), in contradiction to the common notion that generalized edema does not arise after burns of less than 30 % TBSA. The edema in non-injured skin is maximal approximately 1 to 2 days after the injury (27).

Edema promoting mechanisms in non-injured skin are less well investigated than those in burned tissue. The Starling equilibrium describes the filtrative balance across the capillary wall. Included variables are the filtration coefficient, the reflection coefficient for macromolecules and the colloid osmotic pressure (COP) and hydrostatic pressure in plasma and in interstitium. Following larger burns (>30 % TBSA), the capillaries permit egress of somewhat larger macromolecules into uninjured tissues, suggesting a true effect on the capillary reflection coefficient, but less so than in burned areas (19,28). Most likely, inflammatory factors are released from the burn wound to reach uninjured tissues (1,2,14). Nevertheless, the decrease in plasma COP, secondary to loss of circulating protein into injured and uninjured skin must be the most important mechanism (22,29). Crystalloid resuscitation lowers COP further and even an inverse colloid osmotic gradient between plasma and interstitial tissue has been demonstrated up to 12 h post-burn (30).

The non-injured tissue may also have a modified response to an increased net transcapillary filtration of fluid. If healthy animals are overhydrated, there is at first an increase in the interstitial hydrostatic pressure, but with extreme overhydration, the further pressure increase is very modest; in other words, the compliance of the tissue becomes very high (31). The interstitial pressure does not then counterbalance increases in capillary hydrostatic pressure, probably because of matrix changes. One investigation (32) in severely burned patients (>20 % TBSA) showed a standardized pressure on healthy skin could dislocate more fluid for up to 3 weeks, peaking at 6 days. On the other hand, total body water was maximal on day 2, seemingly in parallel with the local edema. This suggests long-lasting changes in the matrix properties of the interstitium, affecting the distribution of fluid. Such changes may also negatively influence lymph flow and resolution of edema (33).

In the kidney, the glomerular filtration threshold is normally around 60 mmHg. A decrease in plasma COP by 10-20 mmHg (30) would imply a decrease in this threshold to around 40-50 mmHg. A satisfactory diuresis is one goal in resuscitation but it should be realized that it can probably be achieved at a lower arterial pressure than in healthy individuals and does not necessarily imply sufficient perfusion of all vascular beds. On the other hand, a low diuresis during resuscitation is taken to indicate lack of fluid and diuretics like furosemide and mannitol are usually contraindicated in this period, not least since they preclude evaluation of rehydration.

In patients, mainly resuscitated with Ringer's acetate, the extracellular water was repeatedly determined as the isohexol space and total body water was assessed as the ethanol space or by bioimpedance (34). Both total body water and the extracellular water peaked one to three days after the burn. One week after the burn, extracellular water was still increased, compared to that in healthy volunteers. No evidence for intracellular fluid accumulation was found. Urinary sodium elimination did not increase until the fourth day post burn, at which time serum plasma sodium concentration was somewhat increased, coinciding with increases in plasma urea and osmolality (35-37).

It should be emphasized that the evaporative losses are considerable after the resuscitation phase and large volumes of glucose solutions or free water by mouth have to be given to avoid hyperosmolality. Minimum amounts of sodium are given to balance for ongoing losses. Closure of wounds can drama-

tically decrease the need for fluid and may predispose for overhydration. In man, sodium-preserving mechanisms are well developed, and are further activated following a trauma, but the capacity to excrete a large overload is limited. After resuscitation, the patient will be in positive sodium balance, whereas, at the same time, there is renal retention of sodium and water and increased excretion of potassium. With uneventful recovery, these changes are reversed. However, sometimes these disturbances persist for weeks or until death (35,38).

Acute renal failure carries a grave prognosis. Its occurrence in the first 5 days is more common after hypotension and myoglobinuria. Late failure is more often associated with sepsis (39) and usually non-anuric. This may coincide with a hyperosmolar state, accentuated by catabolism. An increased osmolar burden may then exceed the renal excretory capacity that seems impaired by tubular dysfunction. It follows that the urine volume cannot be used as the sole indicator of renal function. Furthermore, after the first two days, the urinary output is an unreliable indicator of volume status, as there is often an osmotic diuresis, with excretion of nitrogenous metabolites and glucose.

4.4.3.3. The heart

In burned patients, there may be cardiac dysfunction, appearing within the first 24 h or later. Both the right (40) and the left ventricle (41) and diastolic function (42) can be affected, in spite of normal coronary arteries. Most likely, several mediators in the inflammatory cascades trigger the impairment (as outlined in the introduction). In animal models, there is increased myocardial activity of NF-κB and increased myocardial synthesis of the cytokine TNF alpha within 4 h (9) There is also intracellular calcium overload (43). Notably, plasma concentration of the myocardial enzyme troponin I may increase (44). It follows that even in the early phase, a satisfactory cardiac output may not be achieved by rehydration only and inotropic support is then indicated. The cardiac changes in burns patients are similar to critical illnesses of other etiology, notably sepsis, (45) and are generally reversible.

4.4.3.4. The lung

Crystalloid resuscitation inevitably decreases plasma COP and the question arises whether this increases extravascular lung water. Actually, the lung is relatively protected from a fall in plasma COP and this has been estimated to be about four times less important for filtration than a similar increase in lung capillary hydrostatic pressure (46). It has been argued (47) that pulmonary vasoconstriction protects the lung capillaries initially and overhydration may cause lung edema later, when fluid is mobilized from the tissues. Furthermore, the pulmonary lymph flow is able to compensate for increased transcapillary filtration within wide limits. Indeed, in sheep, following a 40 % skin burn and crystalloid resuscitation, within 48 h, pulmonary lymph flow increased markedly (48) or slightly (49). None of the two studies showed any evidence of increased capillary permeability for proteins. Smoke inhalation (alone nor in conjunction with the standardized burn) did not increase the protein permeability in the lungs, but some conflicting observations exist on this issue (49). Smoke inhalation augmented lung lymph flow markedly, indicating increased filtration of protein free fluid (49).

In clinical practice, overt lung edema is rarely encountered in the first days after a severe burn but is occasionally in a later phase, if sepsis or infective lung complications develop. Thirty-five severely burned and ventilated patients were aggressively resuscitated, by fluid, inotropes and pressor drugs, to an intrathoracic blood volume of >850 mL and to a cardiac index of >3.5 L/min and m^2 (the appropriateness of these goals is not the issue here) (50). Extravascular lung water was measured with a double tracer technique. There was an increase in extravascular lung water only in three measurements out of 140 during the first 48 h.

In a study by Holm et al. (50), 22 patients were considered to have inhaled smoke (soot in airways) even though none displayed increased carboxyhemoglobin concentration. Only one showed evidence of increased extravascular lung water. In several experimental studies, inhalation injury has caused not only increased filtration but increased extravascular water in the lung, but it was argued that the exposure may then have exceeded clinical relevance (50). However, it is common for inhala-

tion injuries to increase the need for resuscitative fluid but this does not imply that more fluid is localized in the lung interstitium and the underlying mechanisms are not clear.

> In the early treatment (e.g. the first 48 h), the main priority in resuscitation appears to be restoration of circulating volume and to obtain a sufficient cardiac output.

Excessive increases in filling pressure should be avoided. It is not easy to determine lung water in clinical practice. Radiographic examination has a high interobserver variability (51) and is not suitable for titration of therapy. Defective oxygenation, as indicated by the need for a higher FiO_2, is not clearly related to increased extravascular lung water (50) but may, more plausibly, as in many other situations in intensive care, reflect atelectasis and other disturbances in ventilation and perfusion. Amelioration can then possibly be achieved by suitable modifications of the ventilatory therapy.

Some methods to assess lung water seem to require further evaluation. In recent years, systems measuring extravascular lung water with a single thermal indicator technique have become clinically available. Only insertion of a specially designed arterial catheter is necessary, provided a central venous line is present. It has been reported that data with a thermal indicator approach differ in some important respects to those obtained by reference methods (52) and further experience will show whether this monitoring will become a useful correlate in clinical routine.

4.4.4. Monitoring and goals of volume resuscitation

The various fluid treatment regimen, like the Parkland formula, are only an initial approximation and often, the volume needed for resuscitation is larger. This calls for monitoring and defined goals but no consensus exists on these matters. Basal monitoring includes heart rate, invasively measured arterial pressure, hourly urine volume, pulse oximetry and measurements of blood gas (including CO-hemoglobin) and lactate. A central venous catheter may be useful for pressure measurements and blood gas sampling. This may be sufficient in less severe cases. It is important to point out that an integrated approach should be applied, including the general clinical status. Sinus tachycardia is usually present (44). Mean arterial pressure is of subordinate use to guide therapy as it usually stays stable or somewhat lowered (47). The hourly urine output remains the most accessible and easily monitored index of resuscitation. It is often targeted at 0.5mL/kg in adults and 1mL/kg in children but as outlined previously and further argued below, this does not *per se* ensure a sufficient perfusion pressure in all tissues. The serum lactate level may be affected by infusion of glucose solutions or adrenergic drugs and reference values differ between laboratories. Nevertheless, lactate is a useful estimate of metabolic status (53,54) and successful therapy is associated with ability to clear elevated serum lactate levels.

In burned patients, the time of the injury is nearly always known and patients are usually treated earlier in the course than are intensive care patients in general. It has been reported that, in non-burned septic patients, early goal directed therapy using the above mentioned variables, is useful to ensure systemic oxygenation after initial resuscitation and hemodynamic stabilization (55). Continuous measurement of mixed venous oxygen saturation with a fiber optic catheter is useful but not always available. The hemoglobin saturation in blood drawn from a central venous catheter may serve as a reasonable surrogate variable (55,56). Values below 65-70 % may indicate impaired peripheral circulation. One caveat is that patients exposed for cyanide, often released in indoor burns and not easily measured, have a spuriously low arteriovenous oxygen difference, due to decreased oxygen utilization.

As previously discussed, cardiac function may be impaired, not only by pre-existing pathology and intercurrent injury but also by the burns injury itself. Cardiac dysfunction may necessitate more intense monitoring, e.g. by a pulmonary artery catheter. Then, measurements of cardiac output are more essential than those of pressures. The typical response to a large burn is an initial decrease in cardiac output (up to 30-60 % of normal) and an increase in systemic resistance (57); the latter mainly owing to increased blood viscosity (24). Successful resuscitation according to the Brooke formula (see below) almost restores cardiac output and plasma volume in 24 h but there is some ongoing destruc-

tion of red cells, precluding normalization of blood volume. Red cell substitution, to a hematocrit of 30-35 %, is best performed after resuscitation. After the first 1-2 days, cardiac output stays above normal reflecting increased metabolism. During resuscitation, pulmonary wedge pressure is usually low to normal. Mean arterial pressure stays normal or is somewhat lowered. Pulmonary artery pressure is initially high but decreases to normal during the first 24 h (47).

Cardiac preload should be a measure of diastolic volume, not pressure, and diastolic dysfunction is not infrequent in severe burns. Echocardiography may be advantageous in cardiac failure (42) and may diagnostic e.g. for hypovolemia, decreased contractility and disturbed relationship between the right and the left ventricle. The ejection fraction is typically increased (up to 0.60-0.85) and is little influenced by fluid loading (47).

In the shock phase, before rehydration, there may be delivery dependent oxygen consumption, as can be expected (58,59). One group reported threshold oxygen delivery values below which such consumption was observed (58). Supranormal values for cardiac index and oxygen delivery after rehydration are linked to survival (53,60,61). This treatment evidently required pulmonary artery monitoring and the improvement was not reflected in arterial pressure, heart rate (53,62) or urine output (62). In non-burned septic patients, however, similar goal directed therapy does not seem to improve, and can even worsen prognosis, possibly because the treatment is not effective in established sepsis (63).

Such goal-directed therapy often implies that large volumes of fluid are given, increasing the overhydration of the tissues. There is no easy solution to the problem. Increased reliance on inotropes and vasopressors in cardiac optimization might be helpful but the effect on outcome of such therapy is insufficiently known. Interestingly, in healthy rats, the alpha-agonist phenylephrine causes NF-κB nuclear translocation, and one study suggested that inflammatory cascades may be enhanced by adrenergic mediators (64). Colloids are probably of limited advantage to decrease edema formation over a longer period (see below). There is a definite need for therapies which reduce the inflammatory impact on the tissues. Plasma exchange has been performed in one study in adult patients who failed to respond to conventional resuscitation. The treatment did not markedly improve the clinical course (65), in contrast to one pediatric study (66) (see below, Pediatric formulae). On the other hand, high doses of intravenous vitamin C given within the initial 24 h have been reported to reduce resuscitation volumes in severely burned patients (67).

Delayed resuscitation, inhalation injury, high voltage injury or extensive full thickness injury increases fluid requirements. Myoglobinemia, e.g. after high voltage injury, necessitates increased resuscitation volume to maintain forced diuresis. It should be pointed out that most burned injuries could be resuscitated using very basic monitoring. It seems important to give priority to swift and sufficient resuscitation (e.g. with regard to urine output and lactate) and later to maintain this state with minimal amounts of fluid. Inotropes and vasopressors should be used with some caution.

4.4.5. The role of macromolecular solutions in resuscitation and later treatment

If a bolus of a colloid solution is infused into a normal subject there will be mobilization of interstitial fluid into the vascular space. At the same time, but more slowly, the infused macromolecules enter the tissues (68). The fluid mobilizing effect is evident also in states of decreased capillary barrier function towards macromolecules but with the enhanced loss of colloid, the volume expansion is less and of shorter duration. Consequently, even in lethal burn injuries with unstable circulation, albumin or dextran infusion temporarily blunts the effects of hypovolemia (69).

Normally, over half of the body's albumin is extravascular and attempts to lastingly increase the circulating fraction by albumin infusion leads to its gradual equilibration with the interstitial compartment. Nevertheless, there is a concentration gradient of albumin and macromolecules, and a COP gradient between plasma and tissues. This is brought about by restriction of the exchange by the semipermeable capillary membranes but also by the lymph flow that clears interstitial macromolecules. In burned patients a new equilibrium is induced with proportionally more interstitial albumin.

In patients with burns > 50 % TBSA, normal serum albumin levels may require the administration of albumin equal to two plasma pools during the first 4-5 days. It has been estimated that one pool will be distributed extravascularly and one is lost within necrotic tissue and, after excision, from the burns wound. Lymphatic recirculation is increased but not enough to keep up with the protein extravasation. Even 3-4 weeks after injury, the fraction of extravascular albumin is increased. Increased catabolism of albumin can be traced for several weeks (70). In burns injuries, proteins other than albumin (e.g. acute phase proteins) contribute proportionally more to plasma COP (29).

If large amounts of albumin are given to increase plasma COP and reabsorb tissue fluid, interstitial COP may eventually increase in proportion to that in plasma. Little edema mobilization can then be expected, which is in line with clinical findings. In pediatric patients serum albumin was maintained above 25 g/L. Compared to controls, there were no significant differences regarding fluid requirements, urine output, ventilatory requirements, length of stay, complication rate or mortality (71). In adult patients with large surface burns aggressive administration of albumin had no effect on total body water or the extracellular space, as measured by bioimpedance or tracer dilution techniques. Even though serum albumin was kept within the normal range, this did not reduce the need for ventilator treatment or diuretics (34).

Thus, maintaining normal serum albumin seems to be without clinical advantage but is associated with high costs. This does not mean that albumin use is of no avail, e.g. in the burned patient with unstable circulation. As discussed below, several fluid regimens use colloids, even early in resuscitation, and have yielded excellent results (see 72). In recent years the notion has been advanced that albumin use in the critically ill is associated with increased mortality (73) but others (74) have refuted this view. The final answer requires further investigations. As with any other drug or plasma substitute, indications and dosage matter and present knowledge concerning albumin is insufficient in these respects.

Artificial colloids, like dextran, hydroxyethyl starch or gelatin can be used to increase the plasma

Colloid formulas	Electrolyte	Colloid	5 % glucose
Moore	See text	Plasma, up to 10 % of body mass in 36 h	See text
Evans	Normal saline 1 mL/kg x % TBSA	Plasma, 1 mL/kg x % TBSA	2000 mL
Brooke	Lactated Ringer's, 1.5 mL/kg x % TBSA	Plasma, 0.5 mL/kg x % TBSA	2000 mL
Slater	Lactated Ringer's, 2000 mL	75 mL/kg, reduced according to response	
Demling	Lactated Ringer's, to maintain urine output at 30 mL/h	Dextran 40 in saline, 2 mL/kg x h for 8 h Fresh frozen plasma, 0.5 mL/h for 18 h, beginning at 8 h postburn	

Table 4.6: Some colloid containing formulas for resuscitation of adult patients. The volumes refer to the first 24 h if not otherwise stated.

COP. In contrast to albumin, these macromolecules have polydisperse molecular weight. The smaller molecules leave the circulation more rapidly and exert a water binding effect in the interstitium. Gelatins, in particular, have a low intravascular persistence. Each colloid has its own profile in terms of kinetics, metabolism, and dependence on renal function and effects on hemostasis. The Scandinavian experience is probably largest with the dextrans that, to a large extent, are eliminated by renal excretion and can be metabolized to water and carbon dioxide. Tissue deposition may be long-lasting with the hydroxyethyl starches, being eliminated by renal excretion.

Some of the reasoning concerning albumin can be applied to these solutions. Thus, Demling et al. (21) demonstrated in animals that the edema in nonburned tissues could be prevented by dextran infusion as long as the COP gradient was augmented. The volume needed for the resuscitation was halved owing to decreased edema formation in nonburned skin. After cessation of colloid infusion, however, this was no longer the case and the need for fluid increased, compared to Ringer controls, so that the total volume of fluid given over the entire observation period was similar. Others (75,76) have similarly reported that starch solutions decreases the edema in unburned skin and the need for resuscitative fluid but the studies were not extended past the resuscitation phase

4.4.6. Resuscitation formulas

4.4.6.1. Colloid resuscitation

Early formulas for resuscitation relied heavily on protein replacement and the burn budget of Moore, initially presented in the 1940-s, utilized plasma, up to 10 % of the body mass in 36 h. External losses, by urine and evaporation, were compensated for by glucose and electrolyte solutions (77). The Evans formula (Table 4.6), presented in 1952, was the first algorithm that calculated the volume of fluid needed from body mass and %TBSA (78). At the Brooke Army Medical Center, the saline was changed to Ringer's lactate and proportionally less plasma was given (Table 4.6). The Slater formula uses lactated Ringer's solution and fresh frozen plasma (Table 4.6). Both fluids are titrated to obtain a satisfactory urine output (79). Dextran 40 in saline, fresh frozen plasma and Ringer's lactate are used in the Demling formula (Table 4.6) (21).

The Mount Vernon formula, which has been used extensively in Britain, was originally based on plasma, 2.5 mL/kg x % TBSA for the first 24 h (see 72). Later, the formula has been based on 5 % albumin.

4.4.6.2. Crystalloid resuscitation

Pruitt and colleagues (80) omitted the plasma from the Brooke formula so that it only contained lactated Ringer's solution (the modified Brooke formula, Table 4.7). Studies at the Parkland Hospital in Dallas indicated that the actual need for Ringer's lactate was 4 mL/kg x % TBSA (Table 4.7). Half of the amount is to be given in the first 8 h (81). This is today the most commonly used algorithm.

Crystalloid formulas	Electrolyte
Modified Brooke	Lactated Ringer's, 2 mL/kg x % TBSA
Parkland	Lactated Ringer's, 4 mL/kg x % TBSA
Monafo	Hypertonic saline, 250 mmol Na$^+$/L Volume to maintain urine output at 30 mL/h. For details, see text

Table 4.7: Some crystalloid formulas for resuscitation of adult patients. The volumes refer to the first 24 h if not otherwise stated.

Hypertonic salt solutions (240-300 mmol/L) are sometimes used in resuscitation, to decrease edema formation. The infusion is targeted at an urine output of 30 mL/h and serum osmolality and sodium are followed (Table 4.7). Normosmolar fluids are used if the serum sodium concentration is above 160 mmol/L (82). It remains controversial whether hypertonic sodium lactate decreases fluid requirements and weight gain (82,83). Furthermore, it has been claimed that such hypertonic resuscitation is associated with a twofold increase in organ failure and a fourfold risk of acute renal failure (84).

The fluid therapy in 83 hospitals in the United States and Canada was reviewed in 1995 (85). The treatment in the first 24 h was predominantly based on crystalloids (just below 90 % of respondents) and the Parkland formula was "often/always" used by 78 %. Colloids were regularly included in the treatment in about 30 %. Hypertonic saline was "often/always" used by 10-15 % of departments. On the second day, colloids were given in about 60 % of departments, in addition to electrolyte and glucose solutions. Wound excision was usually undertaken by days 3 through 5.

4.4.6.3. Pediatric formulas

Children have a proportionally larger body surface area in relation to weight, entailing relatively larger losses from evaporation. The extracellular water compartment is proportionally larger in small children, predisposing for rapid dehydration and circulatory deterioration. On the other hand, children are more vulnerable to fluid overload, with potential worsening of the injury and development

of pulmonary edema or laryngeal swelling necessitating tracheotomy (86). Risk factors as to outcome are age under 4 years, initiation of resuscitation later than 2 hours after the burn, injury by flame and inhalation injury. Several protocols for pediatric resuscitation exist. The Parkland formula can be used, provided that maintenance fluid with glucose (87) is added to the calculated fluid requirements (88,89).

Colloids are often used in pediatric fluid substitution but maintaining a high serum albumin concentration after the resuscitation phase has proven unnecessary (71). Exchange transfusion has been recommended if the patient does not respond favourably to resuscitation, in spite of fluid volumes given exceeding the calculated amount two to three fold. A volume, corresponding to 150 % of the estimated blood volume is exchange transfused, leading to replacement of about 80 % of the child's own blood. This procedure has been shown to normalize fluid resuscitation requirements (66).

4.4.7. Conclusions

Knowledge is increasing concerning the mediators and pathways involved in the inflammatory response to a severe burn injury. The condition requires rapid and adequate resuscitation and carefully titrated fluid therapy, to avoid underhydration and overhydration, the latter potentially jeopardizing tissue nutrition. The resuscitation should be based on the entire clinical picture. The time-honored assessment of hourly diuresis is still important but the measurement of serum lactate seems to convey further information. As the injury may impede the function of several organ systems, notably the heart, more or less invasive monitoring of the central hemodynamics may be of value in selected cases. Crystalloid solutions remain the mainstay of resuscitation and extensive use of colloids has not been demonstrated of advantage.

4.4.8. References

1. Latha B, Babu M. The involvement of free radicals in burn injury: a review. Burns 2001;27:309-17.

2. Zimmerman TJ, Krizek TJ. Thermally induced dermal injury: review of pathophysiologic events and therapeutic intervention. J Burn Care Rehabil 1984;5:193-201.

3. Heughan C, Niinikoski, Hunt TK. Effect of excessive infusion of saline on tissue oxygen transport. Surg Gynecol Obstet 1972;135:257-60.

4. Hunt TK Linsey M, Frislis G et al. The effect of differing ambient oxygen tensions on wound infection. Ann Surg 1974;181:35-39.

5. Zawacki BE. The natural history of reversible burn injury. Surg Gynecol Obst 1974;139:867-72.

6. Ivy ME, Atweh NA, Palmer J et al. Intra-abdominal hypertension and abdominal compartment syndrome in burn patients. J Trauma 2000;49:387-91.

7. Pruitt BJ. Protection from excessive resuscitation: 'pushing the pendulum back'. J Trauma 2000;49:567-68.

8. Ulrich D, Noah EM, Pallua N. Plasma-Endotoxin, Procalcitonin, C-reaktives Protein und Organfunktionen bei Patienten mit schweren Brandverletzungen. Handchir Mikrochir Plast Chir 2001;33:262-266.

9. Maass DL, Hybki DP, White J, Horton JW. The time course of cardiac NF-kappaB and TNF-alpha secretion by cardiac myocytes after burn injury: contribution to burn-related cardiac contractile dysfunction. Shock 2002;17:293-99.

10. Christman JW, Sadikot RT, Blackwell TS. The role of nuclear factor-kappa B in pulmonary diseases. Chest 2000;117:1482-7.

11. Dehne M, Sablotzki A, Hoffmann, A et al. Alterations of acute phase reaction and cytokine production in patients following severe burn injury. Burns 2002;28:535.

12. von Heimburg D, Stieghorst W, Khorram-Sefat R, Pallua N. Procalcitonin—a sepsis parameter in severe burn injuries. Burns 1998;24:745-50.

13. Yowler CJ, Fratianne RB. Current status of burn resuscitation. Clin Plast Surg 2000;27:1-10.

14. Sparkes BG. Immunological responses to thermal injury. Burns 1997;23:106-13.

15. Kelemen JJ, Cioffi WG, Mason AD Effect of ambient temperature on metabolic rate after thermal injury. Ann Surg 1996;223:406-12.

16. Leape LL. Early burn wound changes. J Pediatr Surg 1968;3:292-9.

17. Fox CL, Lasker SE. Fluid and electrolyte alterations in burned monkeys. Ann NY Acad Sci 1968;150:611-7.

18. Monafo WW, Bari WA, Deitz F et al. Increase of sodium in murine skeletal muscle fibers after thermal trauma. Surg Forum 1971;22:51-2.

19. Arturson G. Microvascular permeability to macromolecules in thermal injury. Acta Physiol Scand 1979;463 (Suppl):111-22.

20. Lund T, Onarheim H, Reed RK. Pathogenesis of oedema formation in burn injuries. World J Surg 1992;16:2-9.

21. Demling RH, Kramer GC, Gunther R, Nerlich M. Effect of nonprotein colloid on postburn edema formation in soft tissues and lung. Surgery 1984;95:593-602.

22. Demling RH, Kramer G, Harms B. Role of thermal injury-induced hypoproteinemia on fluid flux and protein permeability in burned and nonburned tissue. Surgery 1984;95:136-44.

23. Onarheim H, Lund T, Reed R. Thermal skin injury: II. Effects on edema formation with lactated Ringer's, plasma and hypertonic saline (2.400 mosmol/l) in the rat. Cirk Shock 1989;27:25-37.

24. Lund T, Bert JL, Onarheim H et al. Microvascular exchange during burn injury. I: A review. Circ Shock 1989;28:179-97.

25. Jelenko C, Jennings WD, O´Kelley WR, Byrd HC. Threshold burning effects on distant microcirculation. Arch Surg 1973; 106: 317-9.

26. Nylander G, Nordström H, Eriksson E. Effects of hyperbaric oxygen on oedema formation after a scald burn. Burns 1984;10:193-6.

27. Demling RH, Kramer G, Harms B. The study of burn wound edema using dichromatic absorptiometry. J Trauma 1978;18:124-8.

28 Carvajal HF, Linares HA, Brouhard BH. Relationship of burn size to vascular permeability changes in rats. Surg Gynecol Obstet 1979;149:193-202.

29. Zetterström H, Arturson G. Plasma oncotic pressure and plasma protein concentration in patients following thermal injury. Acta Anaesth Scand 1980;24:288-94.

30. Pitkänen J, Lund T, Ananderud L, Reed RK. Transcapillary colloid osmotic pressures in injured and non-injured skin of seriously burned patients. Burns 1987;13:198-203.

31. Aukland K, Nicolaysen G. Interstitial fluid volume: local regulatory mechanisms. Physiol Rev 1981;61:556-643.

32. Zdolsek HJ, Lindahl OA, Ängquist KA, Sjöberg F. Non-invasive assessment of intercompartmental fluid shifts in burn victims. Burns 1998;24:233-40.

33. Swartz MA, Kaipainen A, Netti PA et al. Mechanics of interstitial-lymphatic fluid transport: theoretical foundation and experimental validation. J Biomech 1999;32:1297-307.

34. Zdolsek HJ, Lisander B, Jones AW, Sjöberg F. Albumin supplementation during the first week after a burn does not mobilise tissue oedema in humans. Intensive Care Med 2001;27:844-52.

35. Eklund J, Granberg PO, Liljedahl SO. Studies on renal function in burns. Acta Chir Scand 1970;136:627-40.

36. Balogh D, Benzer A, Hackl JM, Bauer M. Sodium balance and osmolarity in burn patients. Int Care Med 1986;12:100-3.

37. Zdolsek HJ. Water physiology in burn victims. Dissertation, Linköping, Dept of Anaesthesiology and Dept of Hand and Plastic Surgery, Linköping University 2000.

38. Planas M, Wachtel T, Frank H, Henderson LW. Characterization of acute renal failure in the burned patient. Arch Intern Med. 1982;142:2087-91.

39. Holm C, Horbrand F, von Donnersmarck GH, Muhlbauer W. Acute renal failure in severely burned patients. Burns 1999;25:171-8.

40. Martyn JA, Snider MT, Szyfelbein SK et al. Right ventricular dysfunction in acute thermal injury. Ann Surg 1980;191:330-5.

41. Reynolds EM, Ryan DP, Sheridan RL, Doody DP. Left ventricular failure complicating severe pediatric burn injuries. J Pediatr Surg 1995;30:264-9.

42. Kuwagata Y, Sugimoto H, Yoshioka T, Sugimoto T. Left ventricular performance in patients with thermal injury or multiple trauma: a clinical study with echocardiography. J Trauma 1992 ;32:158-64.

43. White DJ, Maass DL, Sanders B, Horton JW. Cardiomyocyte intracellular calcium and cardiac dysfunction after burn trauma. Crit Care Med 2002;30:14-22.

44. Murphy JT, Horton JW, Purdue GF, Hunt JL. Evaluation of troponin-I as an indicator of cardiac dysfunction after thermal injury. J Trauma 1998;45:700-4.

45. Bailén MR. Reversible myocardial depression in critically ill, noncardiac patients: A review. Crit Care Med 2002;30:1280-90.

46. Tranbaugh RF, Lewis FR. Crystalloid versus colloid for fluid resuscitation of hypovolemic patients. Adv Shock Res 1983;9:203-16.

47. Baxter CR. Problems and complications of burn shock resuscitation. Surg Clin North Am 1978;58:1313-22.

48. Demling RH, Will JA, Belzer FO.Effect of major thermal injury on the pulmonary microcirculation. Surgery 1978;83:746-51.

49. Soejima K, Schmalstieg FC, Sakurai H et al. Pathophysiological analysis of combined burn and smoke inhalation injuries in sheep.Am J Physiol Lung Cell Mol Physiol 2001; 280(6):L1233-41.

50. Holm C, Tegeler J, Mayr M et al. Effect of crystalloid resuscitation and inhalation injury on extravascular lung water: clinical implications. Chest 2002;121:1956-62.

51. Rubenfeld GD, Caldwell E, Granton J et al. Interobserver variability in applying a radiographic definition for ARDS. Chest 1999;116:1347-53.

52. Wallin CJ, Rosblad PG, Leksell LG. Quantitative estimation of errors in the indicator dilution measurement of extravascular lung water. Int Care Med 1997; 23: 469-75.

53. Holm C, Melcer B, Horbrand F et al. Haemodynamic and oxygen transport responses in survivors and non-survivors following thermal injury. Burns 2000;26:25-33.

54. Jeng JC, Jablonski K, Bridgeman A, Jordan MH. Serum lactate, not base deficit, rapidly predicts survival after major burns. Burns 2002;28:161-6.

55. Rivers E, Nguyen B, Havstad S et al. Early goal-directed therapy in the treatment of severe sepsis and septic shock. N Engl J Med 2001;345:1368-77.

56. Rivers, EP, Ander DS, Powell D. Central venous oxygen saturation monitoring in the critically ill patient. Current Opinion in Critical Care 2001;7:204-11.

57. Pruitt BA Jr. Fluid and electrolyte replacement in the burned patient. Surg Clin North Am 1978;58:1291-1312.

58. Barton RG, Saffle JR, Morris SE et al. Resuscitation of thermally injured patients with oxygen transport criteria as goals of therapy. J Burn Care Rehabil 1997;18:1-9.

59 Holm C, Melcer B, Horbrand F et al. The relationship between oxygen delivery and oxygen consumption during fluid resuscitation of burn-related shock. J Burn Care Rehabil. 2000;21:147-54.

60. Bernard F, Gueugniaud PY, Bertin-Maghit M et al. Prognostic significance of early cardiac index measurements in severely burned patients. Burns 1994;20:529-31.

61. Schiller WR, Bay RC, Garren RL et al. Hyperdynamic resuscitation improves survival in patients with life threatening burns. J Burn Care Rehabil 1997;8:10-6.

62. Dries DJ, Waxman K. Adequate resuscitation of burn patients may not be measured by urine output and vital signs. Crit Care Med 1991;19:327-9.

63. Alia I, Esteban A, Gordo F et al. A randomized and controlled trial of the effect of treatment aimed at maximizing oxygen delivery in patients with severe sepsis or septic shock. Chest 1999;115:453-61.

64. Ballard-Croft C, Maass DL, Sikes P et al. Activation of stress-responsive pathways by the sympathetic nervous system in burn trauma. Shock 2002;18:38-45.

65. Kravitz M, Warden GD, Sullivan JJ, Saffle JR. A randomized trial of plasma exchange in the treatment of burn shock. J Burn Care Rehabil 1989;10:17-26.

66. Stratta RJ, Saffle JR, Kravitz M et al. Exchange transfusion therapy in pediatric burn shock. Circ Shock 1984;12:203-12.

67. Tanaka H, Matsuda T, Miyagantani Y et al. Reduction of resuscitation fluid volumes in severely burned pa-

tients using ascorbic acid administration: a randomized, prospective study. Arch Surg 2000;135:326-31.

68. Berg S, Golster M, Lisander B. Albumin extravasation and tissue washout of hyaluronan after plasma volume expansion with crystalloid or hypooncotic colloid solutions. Acta Anaesthesiol Scand 2002;46:166-72.

69. Shoemaker WC, Matsuda T, State D. Relative hemodynamic effectiveness of whole blood and plasma expanders in burned patients. Surg Gynecol Obst 1977;144:909-14.

70. Birke G, Liljedahl S-O, Plantin L-O, Reizenstein P. Studies on burns. IX. The distribution and losses through the wound of ^{131}I-albumin measured by whole-body counting. Acta Chir Scand 1968;134:27-37.

71. Greenhalgh DG, Housinger TA, Kagan RJ et al. Maintenance of serum albumin levels in pedatric burn patients: a prospective randomised trial. J Trauma 1995;39:67-73.

72. Aharoni A, Abramovici D, Weinberger M et al. Burn resuscitation with a low-volume plasma regimen - analysis of mortality. Burns 1989;15:230-2.

73. Cochrane injuries group. Human albumin administration in critically ill patients: systematic review of randomised controlled trials. Cochrane Injuries Group Albumin Reviewers. BMJ 1998; 317:7153, 235-40.

74. Wilkes MM, Navickis RJ. Patient survival after human albumin administration. Ann Int Med 2001;135:149-64.

75. Guha SC, Kinsky MP, Button B et al. Burn resuscitation: crystalloid versus colloid versus hypertonic saline hyperoncotic colloid in sheep. Crit Care Med 1996;24:1849-57.

76. Brazeal BA, Honeycutt D, Traber LD et al. Pentafraction for superior resuscitation of the ovine thermal burn. Crit Care Med 1995;23:332-9.

77. Moore FD. The body-weight burn budget. Basic fluid therapy for the early burn. Surg Clin North Am 1970;50:1249-65.

78. Evans EI, Purnell OJ, Robinett PW et al. Fluid and electrolyte requirements in severe burns. Ann Surg 1952;135:804-17.

79. Du GB, Slater H, Goldfarb IW. Influences of different resuscitation regimens on acute early weight gain in extensively burned patients. Burns 1991;17:147-50.

80. Pruitt BA Jr, Mason AD Jr, Moncrief JA. Hemodynamic changes in the early postburn patient: the influence of fluid administration and of a vasodilator (hydralazine). J Trauma 1971;11:36-46.

81. Baxter CR, Shires T. Physiological response to crystalloid resuscitation of severe burns. Ann N Y Acad Sci 1968;150:874-94.

82. Monafo WW. The treatment of burn shock by the intravenous and oral administration of hypertonic lactated saline solution. J Trauma. 1970;10:575-86.

83. Gunn ML, Hansbrough JF, Davis JW et al. Prospective, randomized trial of hypertonic sodium lactate versus lactated Ringer's solution for burn shock resuscitation. J Trauma 1989;29:1261-7.

84. Huang PP, Stucky FS, Dimick AR et al. Hypertonic sodium resuscitation is associated with renal failure and death. Ann Surg 1995;221:543-54.

85. Fakhry SM, Alexander J, Smith D et al. Regional and institutional variation in burn care. J Burn Care Rehabil 1995;16:86-90.

86. Coln CE, Purdue GF, Hunt JL. Tracheostomy in the young pediatric burn patient. Arch Surg 1998;133:537-9.

87. Sheridan RL. Burns. Crit Care Med. 2002;30 (Suppl):S500-14.

88. Merrell SW, Saffle JR, Sullivan JJ et al. Fluid resuscitation in thermally injured children. Am J Surg 1986;152:664-9.

89. Graves TA, Cioffi WG, McManus WF et al. Fluid resuscitation of infants and children with massive thermal injury. J Trauma 1988;28:1656-9.

4.5. Volume replacement in the intensive care unit patient

4.5.1. Introduction

Various pathophysiological changes in systemic hemodynamics, organ blood flow, and immune function are present in the intensive care unit (ICU) patient. Adequate management of the underlying insult is required to treat the ICU patient - supportive therapies including optimal nutrition and sufficient volume status appear to be also of importance.

Adequate volume replacement is fundamental for treating the ICU patient. By adequately restoring intravascular fluid volume, organ perfusion may be guaranteed, microcirculatory flow be improved, and subsequently activation of complex series of damaging cascades be avoided (1). It has been reported that in approximately 50 % of septic patients, only adequate volume replacement may reverse hypotension and restore hemodynamics (2). Whether the kind of fluid therapy might modify the vicious cycle induced by hypovolemia or even may influence outcome has not yet been definitely decided.

4.5.2. Specific situation of the intensive care unit patient

Fluid deficits in the ICU patient can occur in the abscence of obvious fluid loss secondary to vasodilation or generalized alterations of the endothelial barrier resulting in diffuse capillary leak. Patients with sepsis/septic shock often show large fluid deficits. Sepsis is characterized by an panendothelial injury with subsequent increased endothelial permeability, loss of proteins, and interstitial edema (3,4). Sepsis is also associated with peripheral vascular paralysis which may result in impaired blood flow regulation to the tissues (5). Thus the complex pathophysiological process associated with sepsis may cause inadequate perfusion and oxygenation subsequently resulting in development of multiple organ dysfunction syndrome (MODS) (6).

The organism tries to compensate hypovolemia-related perfusion deficits by redistribution of flow to vital organs (e.g. heart and brain) resulting in an underperfusion of splanchnic bed, kidney, muscles, and skin (7). Various cytokines and vasoactive substances are of particular importance for deteriorated perfusion in this situation. Activation of the sympathetic nervous system (SNS), the renin-aldosterone-angiotensin system (RAAS), and the antidiuretic system (ADH) are compensatory mechanisms to maintain peripheral perfusion. The principal actions of these systems are to retain water in order to restore intravascular volume deficits, to retain sodium in order to restore the intravascular volume, and to increase the hydrostatic perfusion pressure through vasoconstriction. Although this compensatory neurohumoral activation is beneficial at first, this mechanism becomes deleterious and may be involved in the bad outcome of the critically ill (7). The endothelium does not only function as a passive barrier between the circulating blood and the tissue, endothelial cells are also involved in the regulation of microcirculatory blood flow by producing important regulators of the vascular tone (e.g. prostaglandins, nitric oxide (NO), endothelins, angiotensin II). Blood flow is regulated by a balance between systemic (central) mechanisms (e.g. the autononous nervous system) and other circulating or locally active blood flow regulators.

4.5.3. Guiding volume therapy in the ICU patient

Evaluation of volume deficit and adequate volume therapy remain a challenge. The aim of appropriate monitoring is to avoid sufficient fluid infusion as well as fluid overload. Standard hemodynamic monitoring such as measuring blood pressure and heart rate (HR) are often inaccurate to detect volume deficits or to guide volume therapy. In spite of negative data on the value of pulmonary artery catheters (PAC) in the critically ill, PAC are still widely used for this purpose. However, cardiac filling pressures (e.g. central venous pressure [CVP] and pulmonary artery occlusion pressure [PAOP]) are often misleading surrogates for assessing optimal left ventricular loading conditions. Cardiac filling pressures are influenced by several factors other than blood volume, including alterations in vascular or ventricular compliance and intrathoracic pressure.

Measurement of extravascular lung water (EVLW) and intrathoracic blood volume (ITBV) has been reported to be a more reliable method to monitor volume therapy in this situation (8). By using EVLW and ITBV monitoring, a reduction in ICU and hospital stay was shown and mortality was reduced (9).

Echocardiography, especially transesophageal echocardiography (TEE), appears to be the most specific monitoring instrument to evaluate cardiac filling. Due to its high costs it is not available in every ICU patient. Moreover, TEE is an intermittent rather than a continuous monitoring device.

Perturbations of organ perfusion are thought to be of fundamental importance in the pathogenesis of organ dysfunction in the critically ill (10). The importance of occult hypovolemia for the development of organ perfusion deficits has been supported by several studies (11,12). There is still no optimal routine clinical monitoring to detect perfusion deficits. Hemodynamic parameters such as cardiac output, VO_2, and DO_2 are not regarded to be optimal measures for the adequacy of regional or microcircular perfusion (13). The hypovolemic patient is at risk of experiencing splanchnic hypoperfusion with subsequent development of translocation and systemic inflammatory response syndrome (SIRS) (14). Abnormalities of splanchnic perfusion may coexist with normal systemic hemodynamic and metabolic parameters (14). Non-invasive, continuous tonometry measuring gastric mucosal partial pressure of carbon dioxide (gastric pCO_2) may be an attractive option for diagnosis and monitoring of splanchnic hypoperfusion. In patients undergoing major non-cardiac surgery maintaining hemodynamic stability was no guarantee of an adequate splanchnic perfusion and could not definitely protect against significant postoperative complications (15). Although this monitoring instrument has produced some promising results, it is far from being the new "gold standard" for guiding volume management of the criticially ill (16).

4.5.4. Volume replacement in the ICU patient: what are the conflicts?

Recommendations on the best volume replacement regimen for the ICU patient remain elusive. Although several studies have been focused on the different volume replacement strategies, there are no convincing clear guidelines regarding the choice of fluid for volume replacement in the critically ill. In particular, the choice between colloid and crystalloid solutions continues to generate controversy (17,18,19). In recent years, colloid/colloid discussions have expanded this debate (20).

4.5.4.1. Allogenic blood transfusion

The inherent risk of transmission of viral and immunological diseases has forced us to reduce the use of allogenic blood and blood products. As shown by various studies, reduction in hematocrit and in arterial oxygen content is not deleterious since compensating mechanisms are able to guarantee tissue oxygenation and systemic oxygen transport (21). When non-blood plasma substitutes are used to replace volume deficits, the margin of safety may become compromised especially in patients with significant coronary obstruction. There is an increasing risk of a discrepancy between myocardial oxygen requirements and available subendocardial oxygen supply, which may result in deterioration of myocardial performance. The "optimal" hemoglobin level for patients with sepsis or septic shock is still undetermined. Transfusion of allogenic blood in the patient with an hemoglobin level of 8 to 10 g/dl appears to be without benefit with regard to tissue perfusion or oxygena-

tion (22). Elevating hemoglobin levels higher than 7 to 10 mg/d has been also shown to be without any benefit in outcome in ICU patients (22). Blood transfusions may even have detrimental effects on organ perfusion, oxygenation (e.g. of the splanchnic circulation), and immune function (23, 24). Thus it appears generally accepted that the use of blood/blood products should be restricted to those cases requiring an increase in hemoglobin or treatment of coagulopathy (25,26).

4.5.4.2. Crystalloids versus colloids

When compared with colloids, crystalloids are frequently preferred for volume replacement because they are inexpensive and are almost free of side effects (27).

■ Coagulation

Crystalloids are mainly considered not to affect hemostasis. Interest has recently been focused on the influence of crystalloids on hemostasis. There is convincing evidence that use of crystalloids have a substantial influence on coagulation. Ruttmann et al (28) and Ng et al (29) showed that in vivo dilution with crystalloids resulted in significant enhancement of coagulation. The reason for the hypercoagulable state appears to be an imbalance between naturally occuring anticoagulants and activated procoagulants with a reduction in antithrombin III probably being the most important (28). Others have also documented hypercoagulability with the use of crystalloids (30). This increase in coagulation seems to be independent from the type of crystalloid that has been used (30). An early study reported that the increase in coagulation in patients in whom crystalloids were given during surgery was associated with an increased incidence of deep vein thrombosis (31).

■ Organ dysfunction

The use of saline solution (SS), particularly in large doses, has been shown to be associated with severe (hyperchloremic) acidosis (32). The importance of this type of acidosis for organ function is far from being clear. In healthy volunteers receiving either Ringer's solution (RL) or SS, 10 patients in the SS group experienced abdominal discomfort whilst only one did of the LR group (33). There is increasing evidence that hyperchloremic acidosis may impair end organ perfusion: hyperchloremia has been shown to possess negative effects on renal blood flow and glomerular filtration rate (GFR) (34).

■ Tissue edema

Development of (pulmonary) edema may be one complication of volume replacement in the critically ill especially when large amounts of volume are necessary to stabilize hemodynamics (figure 4.6). Extracellular fluid accumulation appears to be a major factor in the pathogenesis of organ failure. Elements which contribute to tissue edema formation are:

- 1. venous congestion
- 2. reduced colloid osmotic pressure (COP)
- 3. arteriolar vasodilation/venous vasoconstriction
- 4. disorganisation of interstitial matrix
- 5. increased endothelial permeability and
- 6. lymphatic dysfunction.

Apart from an increased hydrostatic pressure, a low COP may predispose to (pulmonary) edema. Colloids may have some advantages because they do not lower COP, whereas crystalloids reduce COP, potentially predisposing the patient to the development of pulmonary and/or systemic edema. In contrast to use of crystalloids, colloid volume replacement appears not to be associated with edema formation: in a study in 26 mostly septic patients, in whom either colloids or crystalloids were infused on the ICU, patients receiving 0.9 % saline showed a higher incidence of pulmonary edema than patients treated with a HES-preparation (35).

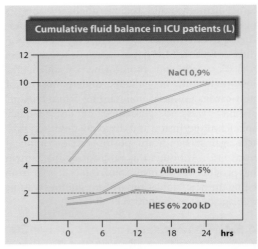

Figure 4.6: Volume therapy with exclusively either albumin HES 200/0.5 or crystalloids (saline solution). Approximately 10 L of crystalloids are necessary to stablize hemodynamics of the hypovolemic patient.

By contrast, the concept of "leaky capillaries" has been used as an argument against the use of colloids and pro crystalloids. The rational is that colloids also leak out of the capillaries into the interstitial space (ISS), increase COP in the interstitium and so drag water in the ISS resulting in exacerbation of interstitial edema. Whether all colloids are equal in this situation has been extensively discussed. There is experimental and clinical evidence that starch preparations with a narrow range medium molecular weight (200 kD) are more effective in avoiding or reducing capillary permeability edema than other preparations (36). Use of albumin is not helpful in this situation (37).

In patients with altered lung function (e.g. in ARDS), although (interstitial) fluid overload is undesired, it often cannot be avoided in septic patients showing extensive inflammation and capillary leak. In this situation, a restrictive volume replacement regimen seems to be promising (38). It is important to stress that the consequences of pulmonary fluid overload can easily be compensated by modern ventilation regimen; hypovolemia-induced MODS, however, is incurable and often results in death.

■ Microcirculation

Compared to colloids, even a massive crystalloid resuscitation alone is less likely to achieve adequate restoration of (microcirculatory) blood flow

(40,41). In a septic animal experiment greater capillary luminal area associated with less endothelial swelling and less parenchymal injury was shown with colloid infusion (pentastarch) than with Ringer's lactate (40). In patients undergoing major abdominal surgery, the influence of a new, third-generation HES (HES 130/0.4) on tissue pO_2 was compared to patients who received only saline solution for volume replacement using flexible minimal-invasive microsensoric pO_2-catheters (42). Although systemic hemodynamics and oxygenation data were kept unchanged from baseline and were similar in both groups within the entire study period, tissue pO_2 increased significantly in the HES-treated patients (maximum +59 %), whereas it decreased in the RL group (maximum -23 %). Thus intravascular volume replacement with HES 130/0.4 improved tissue oxygenation during and after major surgical procedures compared to a crystalloid-based volume replacement strategy.

4.5.4.3. Colloids versus colloids

The available colloids differ with regard to their physico-chemical and pharmacological characteristics and subsequently in their clinical effects and side-effects in the ICU patient.

■ Coagulation

The critically ill patient is at risk of developing coagulation abnormalities at different levels. All agents used for volume replacement therapy lower the concentration of clotting proteins by means of hemodilution. Some colloids appear to possess some additional specific effects on hemostasis.

Albumin is often preferred especially in the ICU patient with compromised hemostasis because it is considered to have no negative effects on coagulation. However, an in vitro study using serial hemodilution (11 %, 25 %, 33 %, 50 %, 75 %) and thrombelastography (TEG) showed that albumin may also produce early and profound hypocoagulable effects (42). Dextrans are well known to negatively influence hemostasis most likely due to a reduction in von Willebrand factor (vWf) or to impairment of platelet function (43).

Gelatins have been considered to be without major negative influence on the coagulation process, although in an in vitro study, however, platelet aggregation was significantly inhibited by two gelatin preparations (polygeline, and succinylated gelatin) (44).

Use of hydroxyethylstarch for volume replacement has been shown to result in abnormal hemostasis and subsequent bleeding complications (45). Most reports on deteriorated hemostasis with starches originate from administration of first-generation high-molecular weight (HMW) - HES (hetastarch). Infusion of this HES specification may result in a type I von Willebrand-like syndrome with reduced factor VIII coagulant activity, and decreased von Willebrand's factor antigen and factor VIII-related ristocetin cofactor. HES with lower molecular weight (LMW-HES) appears to influence coagulation significantly less than HMW-HES (46). Summarizing the controversy of the "HES and coagulation" debate it has been confirmed by several human studies that modern HES preparations with a low MW and a low MS can be safely used without risk of significantly disturbing hemostasis and inducing severe bleeding tendency (46). A completely new, third-generation HES preparation with a MW of 130 kD, a MS of 0.4, and a C2/C6 ratio of >8 has an improved physico-chemical profile. The maximum daily dose with the substance has been enlarged from 33 mL/kg to 50 mL/kg. This kind of HES is associated with almost no negative effects on the coagulation process (47).

■ Renal function

Impaired renal function in the ICU patient may be a problem especially when using (synthetic) colloids. The effects of different volume replacement regimens on renal function in ICU patients are controversially discussed (table 4.8) (48-52). Gelatins and albumin appear to be without significant damaging effects. Elimination of HES molecules varies with molecular weight (Mw) and, most importantly, with the molar substitution (MS). Large HES molecules are split by hydrolytic cleavage by alpha-amylase. The smaller HES molecules (and also gelatin molecules) are eliminated by glomerular filtration. Some histological studies have shown reversible swelling of tubular cells of the kidneys after administration of HES, gelatins and dextrans, which appears to be most likely due to reabsorption of macromolecules. Swelling of tubular cells may result in tubular obstruction and medullar ischemia and, subsequently, in development of acute renal failure. Glomerular filtration of hyper-

Author/ year (Reference)	substance no. of patients	pro/retro rand/d-b	kind of patients	aim	renal function prior to study	conclusion
London (1989) (48)	10 % HES 260/0.45 (n=50) 5 % HA (n=44)	pro rand	ICU after cardiac surgery	maintain CI >2.0 l/min/m^2	normal kidney function	creatinine + urine output: no differences **outcome: no differences**
Stockwell (1992) (49)	5 % HA (n=226) gelatin (n=249)	pro rand	ICU patients	general volume replacement	not known	ARF: no differences (HA n=3; gelatin n=5) **outcome: no differences**
Boldt (1998) (50)	10 % HES 200/0.5 (n=150) 20 % HA (n=150)	pro rand	ICU patients trauma and sepsis	PCWP 12-15 mmHg	normal creatinine: 1.0-1.9 mg/dl	creatinine + urine output: no differences **outcome: no differences**
Allison (1999) (51)	6 % HES 250/0.45 (n=24) gelatin (n=21)	pro rand	ICU trauma patients	not defined	not known	creatinine + urine output: no differences **outcome: not shown**
Schortgen (2001) (52)	6 % HES 200/0.62 (n=65) gelatin (n=64)	pro rand multi-center	sepsis/septic shock ICU patients	fixed dose	elevated creatinine levels	HES: more ARF HES 42 %; Gelatine: 23 % **outcome: no differences**

Table 4.8: Studies comparing effects of different volume replacement regimen on renal function in ICU patients. pro: prospectively; rand: randomized; HES: hydroxethyl starch; HA: human albumin; d-b: double-blind; CI: cardiac index; ARF: acute renal failure; ICU: intensive care unit.

oncotic molecules from colloids causes a hyperviscose urine and stasis of tubular flow resulting in obstruction of tubular lumen. In a retrospective study in brain-dead kidney donors in whom HES with a high MS (0.62) was infused, "osmotic-nephrosis-like lesions" were documented (53). These lesions had no negative effects on graft function or serum creatinine 3 and 6 months after transplantation. In a multicenter study of 129 ICU patients with sepsis or septic shock the effects of volume therapy on kidney function with either a HES preparation with a high MS (200/0.62) or gelatin was assessed (52). The median cumulative volume replacement was 31mL/kg with HES and 43mL/kg with gelatin. Acute renal failure (defined as a two-fold increase in serum creatinine concentration or need for renal replacement therapy) developed in 27 of the HES-treated patients (42 %) and in 15 of the gelatin-infused patients (23 %) (p<0.028). Unfortunately, the two volume groups showed different creatinine levels prior to the start of volume therapy: median serum creatinine concentrations was 143 µmol/l in the HES-treated patients and 114 µmol/l in the gelatin-treated patients. Compared with the gelatin-group, use of the

slowly degradable HES preparation (HES 200/0.62) was an independent risk factor for the occurrence of ARF. Inspite of a higher incidence of ARF in the HES-treated patients, mortality was not significantly different between the two groups.

HES preparations with different physico-chemical characteristics (especially lower MS) do not appear to impair renal function in patients with normal kidney function: long-term (over 5 days) use of HES 200/0.5 in critically ill ICU patients did not have negative effects on renal function compared to a control group in whom albumin was administered (50). Promising results have been shown with the third-generation, rapidly degradable HES preparation: in patients with moderate-to-severe kidney dysfunction 400mL of HES 130/0.4 was not associated with further deterioration of kidney function (54).

■ Immune system

Infection, trauma, or critical illness initiate an inflammatory cascade which leads to an activation of regulatory mechanisms aimed to control the intensity of the inflammatory response. In addition to improve hemodynamics, optimization of the patient's intravascular volume status may have important effects on immune response (55). The influence of a specific fluid therapy, particularly of synthetic colloids, on immune function is only rarely studied. The sequelae of HES on endothelial cell activation was studied experimentally by Collis et al (56) using endothelial cell cultures (human umbilical vein endothelial cells [HUVECs]). Expression of the adhesion ligand E-selectin on lipopolysaccharide-stimulated endothelial cells was not influenced by HES. The authors suggested a possible beneficial role of HES by inhibiting endothelial activation: HES may be involved in preventing neutrophil adhesion during the inflammatory process. In animals undergoing severe hemorrhage, levels of inflammatory cytokines (interleukin-6) were not negatively affected by HES (57). The authors concluded that immunodepression after hemorrhage depends more on the severity of hemorrhage than on the resuscitation regimen. In an in vitro study, T-cell activation and mitogenic responses were not inhibited in the presence of dextran, gelatin or HES indicating no immunodepression by colloidal resuscitation fluids (58). The time- and dose-dependent generation of a chemotactic cytokine was not affected by the presence of HES (59). HES alone did not induce cytokine generation nor were human monocytes chemotaxis and spontaneous migration changed (59). Circulating endothelial-derived adhesion molecules are less increased in septic patients treated with HES 200/0.5 than after infusion of albumin (Figure 4.7) indicating preservation of endothelial function by HES (60). Information of the influence of other plasma substitutes on the immune system is widely incomplete.

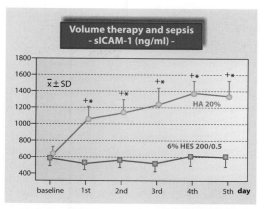

Figure 4.7: Plasma levels of soluble intercellular adhesion molecule-1 (sICAM-1) in septic intensive care unit patients whom received exclusively human albumin 20 % or HES 200/0.5 over 5 days to stabilize hemodynamics.

4.5.5. Does a specific volume replacement strategy affect outome of the ICU patient?

In published meta-analyses comparing colloids with crystalloids the conclusions vary. Some studies provide false hopes about the importance of a certain volume replacement regimen ("Resuscitation with colloids was associated with... four extra deaths for every 100 patients resuscitated." (18)). In a systematic review on crystalloids versus colloids in fluid resuscitation, 17 relevant studies out of 105 articles from 1966 to 1996 were identified (58). Pulmonary edema, mortality and length of stay were evaluated. In the subgroup "Critical Care" only 3 studies were analysed - two were over 15 years old and one study from 1994 included (non-ICU) patients undergoing interleukin-2-based therapy for metastatic cancer and volume therapy. None of the analysed factors (outcome, mortality) were significantly influenced by either of the volume replacement regimens. In an another Cochrane Review-based meta-analysis the effects on mortality of colloids compared to crystalloids for fluid resuscitation were assessed (60). 26 trials comparing crystalloids with different kinds of colloids, 9 trials comparing colloids prepared in hypertonic crystalloids with isotonic crystalloids, and 3 trials comparing hypertonic crystalloids with colloids were included. There was no evidence that resuscitation with colloids reduces the risk of death in patients with trauma, burns and following surgery.

It has been questioned whether meta-analyses focusing on outcome are appropriate instruments to examine the value of different fluid therapies in the critically ill (60,61), because mortality was never an end point of any of the underlying studies. New concepts about critical care, e.g. the role of inflammation, immunological aspects, and organ function may shed new light on this problem. Whether a randomised control trial comparing different solutions that is strictly focused on outcome is substantial in the ICU setting has been doubted. It would require over 6,500 patients with comparable underlying diseases who are very similarly treated to detect excess mortality of 4 % (60). In view of the complexity of the underlying disease of the ICU patient, administration of one single substance is unlikely to significantly modify outcome. At present, it appears to be a myth to believe that a certain fluid type may save somebody's life on the ICU.

4.5.6. Conclusions

Volume replacement in the ICU patient requires understanding of the pathophysiology of the underlying disease, the physiology of fluid compartments and volume of distribution, and the knowledge of the pharmacokinetics of the different solutions for volume replacement.

Adequate volume replacement appears to be a cornerstone for managing the ICU patient because restoration of microcirculatory blood flow is an essential key to avoid tissue ischemia or reperfusion injury. Fluid restriction in the hypovolemic patient is a prescrition for development of a clinical disaster.

> The "dry and die, wet and survive" philosophy cannot generally be recommended, but the risk of development of vital organ hypoperfusion in the hypovolemic patient has to be considered carefully when plannig to embark on the strategy of keeping the patient dry.

Merits and demerits of each solution for volume replacement have to be considered carefully including the effects on hemostasis, renal function, and other organ systems. Because of the important differences between individual colloids, it appears not to be appropriate to summarize all colloids in a "colloid group". Albumin is still often used on ICUs, however, in todays climate of cost consciousness and cost containment alternatives to the high-priced albumin are of interest. Replacing albumin by an appropriate modern synthetic colloid can markedly reduce ICU cost. The safety and effectiveness of modern synthetic colloids are well documented and several studies concluded that albumin can be safely abandoned in the treatment of the hypovolemic ICU patient.

> No specific recommendation can be made at present with regard to the choice of fluid and outcome. Most studies were not primarily focused on outcome, outcome was even not shown in several studies, or the studies did not include enough ICU patients to determine the best volume replacement strategy.

What endpoints should be chosen when the "ideal" volume replacement strategy is assessed? Although often used, "clinical signs" of hypovolemia are nonspecific and insensitive. We need better monitoring technologies that will help to guide our volume therapy and improved "point-of-care" markers that will help us to better assess whether our volume therapy is appropriate in the ICU patient. More information on changes in regional perfusion, microcirculation and inflammation especially with different serial, long-term volume replacement strategies is necessary.

4.5.7. Message

- Sufficient volume replacement is a prerequisite in treating the intensive care unit (ICU) patient.

- Exclusive use of large amounts of crystalloids is associated with the risk of interstitial edema formation and impaired microperfusion.

- To keep the ICU patient dry and to use more catecholamines may result in catastrophic organ perfusion deficits and in the development of multiple organ failure (MOF).

- Theoretical benefits of albumin have not been supported by clinical studies. For treating the hypovolemic ICU patient, albumin can be avoided without risk.

- Modern synthetic colloids are cheap and effective plasma substitutes.

- A modern, third-generation, hydroxyethyl-starch solution (HES 130/0.4) appears to avoid negative effects of other HES specifications.
- There seems to be no convincing advantage of either solution with regard to outcome.

4.5.8. References

1. Gosling P, Bascom JU, Zikria BA (1996) Capillary leak, oedema and organ failue: breaking the triad. Care of the Critically Ill 12:191-197

2. Task Force of the American College of Critical Care Medicine, Society of Critical Care Medicine (1999) Practice parameters for hemodynamic support of sepsis in adult patients in sepsis. Crit Care Med 27: 639-660

3. Thijs LG (1995) Fluid therapy in septic shock. In: Sibbald WJ, Vincent JL (eds): Clinical trials for the treatment of sepsis. Update in Intensive Care and Emergency Medicine, vol 19. Springer, Berlin Heidelberg New York, 167-190

4. Fleck A, Raines G, Hawker F, Trotter J, Wallace PI, Ledingham IM (1985) Increased vascular permeability: a major cause of hypalbuminaemia in disease and injury. Lancet i:781-784

5. Natanson C (1994) Selected treatment strategies for septic shock based on proposed mechansims of pathogenesis. Ann Intern Med 120:771-783

6. Pittard AJ, Hawkins WJ, Webster NR (1994) The role of the microcirculation in the multi-organ dysfunction syndrome. Clin Intensive Care 5:186-190

7. Turnbull AV, Little RA (1993) Neuro-hormonal regulation after trauma. Circulating cytokines may also contribute to an activated sympathetic-adrenal control. In: Vincent JL (ed) Update in Intensive Care and Emergency Medicine. Springer, Berlin Heidelberg New York Tokyo, pp 574-581

8. Sakka SG, Bredle DL, Reinhardt K, Meier-Hellmann A (1999) Comparison between intrathoracic blood volume and cardiac filling pressures in the early phase of hemodynamic instability of patients with sepsis or septic shock. J Crit Care Med 14:78-83

9. Mitchell JP, Schuller D, Calandrino FS, Schuster DP (1992) Improved outcome based on fluid management in critically ill patients requiring pulmonary artery catheterization. Am Rev Respir Dis 145:990-998

10. Pittard AJ, Hawkins WJ, Webster NR (1994) The role of the microcirculation in the multi-organ dysfunction syndrome. Clin Intensive Care 1994; 5:186-190

11. Fiddian-Green RG (1990) Gut mucosal ischaemia during cardiac surgery. In: Taylor K, ed. Sem Cardiovasc Surg. Philadelphia: WB Saunders, 1-11

12. Mythen MG, Webb AR (1994) The role of gut mucosal hypoperfusion in the pathogenesis of postoperative organ dysfunction. Intensive Care Med 20:203-209

13. Gutierrez G, Bismar H, Dantzker DR, et al (1992) Comparison of gastric intramucosal pH with measures of oxygen transport and consumption in critically ill patients. Crit Care Med 20:451-457

14. Mythen MG, Webb AR (1995) Perioperative plasma volume expansion reduces the incidence of gut mucosal hypoperfusion during cardiac surgery. Ann Surg 130:423-429

15. Marik PE, Iglesias J, Marini B (1997) Gastric intramucosal pH changes after volume replacement with hydroxyethyl starch or crystalloid in patients undergoing elective abdominal aortic aneurysm repair. J Crit Care 12:51-55

16. Bams JL, Mariani MA, Groneveld ABJ (1999) Predicting outcome after cardiac surgery: comparison of global haemodynamic and tonometric variables. Br J Anaesth 82:33-37

17. Liepert DJ, Pearl RG (1999) Resuscitation and lung water: crystalloid versus colloid. In: Prough DS (ed): Fluids and electrolytes. Problems in Anesthesia 11:447-457

18. Schierhout G, Roberts I (1998) Fluid resuscitation with colloids or crystalloids in critically ill patients: a systematic review of randomised trials. BMJ 316:961-964

19. Velanovich V (1989) Crystalloid versus colloid fluid resuscitation: a meta-analysis of mortality. Surgery 105:65-71

20. Cochrane Injuries Group Albumin Reviewers (1998) Human albumin administration in critically ill patients: systematic review of randomised controlled trials. BMJ 317: 235-239

21. Spahn DR, Leone BJ, Reves JG, Pasch T (1994) Cardiovascular and coronary physiology of acute isovolemic hemodilution: a review of nonoxygen-carrying and oxygen-carrying solutions. Anesth Analg 78:1000-1021

22. Hebert P, Wells G, Blajchman A, et al (1999) A multicenter randomized, controlled clinical trial of transfusion requirements in critical care. N Engl J Med 340:409-417

23. Marik P, Sibbald W (1993) Effect of stored-blood transfusion in oxygen delivery in patients with sepsis. JAMA 269:3024-3029

24. Landers DF, Hill GE, Wong KC, Fox IJ (1996) Blood transfusion-induced immunomodulation. Anesth Analg 82:187-204

25. Goodnough LT, Brecher ME, Kanter MH, AuBuchon JP (1999) Transfusion medicine. First of two parts - blood transfusion. N Engl J Med 340:438-447

26. Goodnough LT, Brecher ME, Kanter MH, AuBuchon JP (1999) Transfusion medicine. Second of two parts - blood conservation. N Engl J Med 340:525-533

27. Hillman K, Bishop G, Bristow P (1997) The crystalloid versus colloid controvery: present status. Balliere`s Clin Anaesth 11:1-13

28. Ruttmann TG, James MFM, Finlayson J (2002) Effects on coagulation of intravenous crystalloid or colloid in patients undergoing peripheral vascular surgery. Br J Anaesth 89:226-230

29. Ng KFJ, Lam CCK, Chan LC (2002) In vivo effect of haemodilution with saline on coagulation: a randomized controlled trial. Brit J Anaesth 2002; 88:475-480

30. Boldt J, Haisch G, Suttner S, Kumle B, Schellhaas A (2002) Are lactated Ringer`s solution and normal saline solution equal with regard to coagulation? Anesth Analg 94:378-384

31. Janvrin SB, Davies G, Greenhalgh RM (1980) Postoperative deep vein thrombosis caused by intravenous fluids during surgery. Brit J Surg 1980; 67:690-693

32. Mathes DD, Morell RC, Rohr MS (1997) Dilutional acidosis: is it a real clinical entity? Anesthesiology 86:501-503.

33. Williams EL, Hildebrannd KL, McCormick SA, Bedel MJ (1999) The effect of intravenous lactated Ringer`s solution versus 0-9 % sodium chloride on serum osmolality in human volunteers. Anesth Analg 88:999-1003

34. Wilcox CS (1983) Regulation of renal blood flow by plasma chloride. J Clin Invest 71:726-735

35. Rackow EC, Falk, Fein A, Siegel JS, Packman MI, Haupt MT, Kaufman BS, Putman D (1983) Fluid resuscitation in circulatory shock: A comparison of the cardiorespiratory effects of albumin, hetastarch, and saline solutions in patients with hypovolemic and septic shock, Crit Care Med 11: 839-850

36. Yeh Tjr, Pamar JM, Reseyka IM (1992) Limiting edema in neonatal cardiopulmonary bypass with narrow range molecular weight hydroxyethyl starch. J Thorac Cardiovasc Surg 14:659

37. Boldt J, v Bormann B, Kling D, Börner U, Mulch J, Hempelmann G (1985) Colloidosmotic pressure and extravascular lung water after extracorporeal circulation. Herz 10:366-375

38. Schuster DP (1995) Fluid management in ARDS: "keep them dry" or does it matter? Intensive Care Med 21: 101-103

39. Funk W, Baldinger V (1995) Microcirculatory perfusion during volume therapy. Anesthesiology 82: 975-982

40. Wang P, Hauptman JG, Chaudry IH (1990) Hemorrhage produces depression in microvascular blood flow which persist despite fluid resuscitation. Circ Shock 32: 307-318

41. Lang K, Boldt J, Suttner S, Haisch G (2001) Colloids versus crystalloids and tissue oxygen tension in patients undergoing major abdominal surgery. Anesth Analg 93:405-409

42. Tobias MD, Wambold D, Pilla MA, Greer F (1998) Differential effects of serial hemodilution with hydroxyethyl starch, albumin, and 0.9 % saline on whole blood coagulation. J Clin Anesth 8: 366-371

43. Halonen P, Linko K, Myllylä G (1987) A study of haemostasis following use of high doses of hydroxyethyl starch 120 and dextran in major laparotomies. Acta Anaesthesiol Scand 31:320-4

44. Evans PA, Glenn JR, Heptinstall S, Madira W (1998) Effects of gelatin-based resuscitation fluids on platelet aggregation. Br J Anaesth 81: 198-292, 1998

45. Warren BB, Durieux ME (1997) Hydroxyethylstarch: safe or not? Anesth Analg 84: 206-212

46. deJonge E, Levi M (2001) Effects of different plasma substitutes on blood coagulation: a comparative review. Crit Care Med 29:1261-1267

47. Haisch G, Boldt J, Krebs C, Kumle B, Suttner S, Schulz A (2001) The influence of intravascular volume therapy with a new hydroxyethyl starch preparation (6 % HES 130/0.4) on coagulation in patients undergoing major abdominal surgery. Anesth Analg 92:565-571

48. London MJ, Ho SJ, Triedman JK, et al. A randomized clinical trial of 10 % pentastarch (low molecular weight hydroxyethyl starch) versus 5 % albumin for plasma volume expansion after cardiac operations. J Thorac Cardiovasc Surg 1989; 97:785-797

49. Stockwell MA, Scott A, Day A, Soni N. Colloid solutions in the critically ill. A randomised comparison of albumin and polygeline. 2. Serum albumin concentration and incidences of pulmonary oedema and acute renal failure. Anaesthesia 1992; 47:7-9

50. Boldt J, Müller M, Mentges D, Papsdorf M, Hempelmann G (1998) Volume therapy in the critically ill: is there a difference? Intensive Care Med 24:28-36

51. Allison KP, Gosling P, Jones S, et al. Randomized trial of hydroxyethyl starch versus gelatine for trauma resuscitation. J Trauma 1999; 47:1114-1121

52. Schortgen F, Lacherade JC, Bruneel F, Cattaneo I, Hemery F, Lemaire F, Brochard L (2001) Effects of hydroxyethylstarch and gelatin on renal function in severe sepsis: a multicentre randomised study. Lancet 357:911-916

53. Legendre C, Thervet E, Page B, Percheron A, Noel LH, Kreis H (1993) Hydroxyethyl starch and osmotic-nephrosis-like lesions in kidney transplantation. Lancet 342:248-249

54. Jungheinrich C, Scharf R, Wargenau M, Bepperling F, Baron JF (2002) The pharmacokinetics and tolerability of an intravenous infusion of the new hydroxyethyl-starch 130/0.4 (6 %, 500mL) in mild-to-severe renal impairment. Anesth Analg 95:544-551

55. Wilson MA, Chou MC, Spain DA, Downard PJ, Qian Q, Cheadle WG, Garrison RN (1996) Fluid resuscitation attenuates early cytokine mRNA expression after peritonitis. J Trauma 41:622-627

56. Collis RE, Collins PW, Gutteridge CN, Faul A, Newland AC, Williams DM, Webb AR (1994) The effect of hydroxyethyl starch and other plasma volume substitutes on endothelial cell activation; an in vitro study. Intensive Care Med 20:37-41

57. Schmand J, Ayala A, Chaudry IH (1994) Effects of trauma, duration of hypotension, and resuscitation regimen on cellular immunity after hemorrhagic shock. Crit Care Med 22:1076-1083

58. Sillett HK, Whicher JT, Trejdowiewicz LK (1998) Effects of resuscitation fluids on T cell immune response. Br J Anaesth 1998; 81:242-243

59. Eastlund DT, Douglas MS, Choper JZ (1992) Monocyte chemotaxis and chemotactic cytokine release after exposure of hydroxyethyl. Transfusion 32:855-860

60. Boldt J, Müller M, Heesen M, Martin K, Hempelmann G (1996) Influence of different volume therapies and pentoxifylline infusion on circulating soluble adhesion molecules in critically ill patients. Crit Care Med 24:385-391

58. Choi P, Yip G, Quinonez L, Cook D (1999) Crystalloids versus colloids in fluid resuscitation: A systematic review. Crit Care Med 27:200-210

59. Alderson P, Schierhout G, Roberts I, Brunn F (2002) Colloids versus crystalloids for fluid resuscitation in critically ill patients (Chochrane Review). The Cochrane Library, Issue 3

60. Webb AR (1999) Crystalloid or colloid resuscitation. Are we any wiser? Crit Care 3:R25-R28

61. Astiz ME, Rackow EC (1999) Crystalloid-colloid controversy revisited. Crit Care Med 27:34-35

4.6. Volume replacement in neurosurgery

Perioperative treatment of neurosurgical patients differs from that of other surgical therapies as the brain and spinal cord represent the target organ for both anesthesiologists *and* neurosurgeons. In patients with neurological diseases one or more of the following pathophysiological processes may be relevant:

- *space occupying lesions* (e.g. tumor, abscess, or hematoma)
- *edema formation*
- *increased intracranial pressure*
- *dysfunction of cerebral and spinal blood flow* (e.g. by hypovolemia, spinal shock syndrome, or cerebral vasospasm).

As a consequence of the low ischemic and hypoxic tolerance of the brain and spinal cord perioperative neuroanesthetic concepts are required to allow for optimal neurosurgical or neuroradiological conditions while minimizing hypoxic-ischemic neuronal damage and/or resuscitating injured neuronal tissue.

Perioperative fluid-management is essential in prevention and therapy of hypoxic-ischemic complications. The classical approach of fluid restriction to avoid brain edema formation was frequently associated with hypovolemia and in turn arterial hypotension. However, according to the *Traumatic Coma Data Bank* arterial hypotension and hypovolemia are most relevant factors in the generation of secondary brain damage. Therefore, the current approach of volume replacement in neurosurgical patients focuses at the maintenance of normovolemia or mild hypervolemia (1).

4.6.1. Physiologic principles

The intention of any perioperative fluid therapy is to optimize the plasma volume, the cerebral perfusion pressure and the microcirculation without generation of tissue edema. An optimal fluid therapy is based on the knowledge of the anatomy and function of biological membranes and the principles of fluid exchange between the extracellular and the intracellular compartment.

Total body water consists of the *extracellular* and the *intracellular* fluid volume separated by a semipermeable membrane. These biological membranes between the extracellular and the intracellular space are easily permeable for water. In contrast, ions permeate slowly and larger molecules hardly ever diffuse through the membrane. The extracellular compartment consists of the *plasma volume (intravascular space)* and the *interstitial fluid volume*. In peripheral tissues the fluid exchange between both compartments is governed by the hydrostatic and the oncotic pressure. Water, ions, and, small molecules can easily pass the endothelial cell layer of the capillaries through gap junctions, while this structure is rather impermeable for larger molecules (e.g. albumin and synthetic colloids) (figure 4.8). Therefore, the precapillary hydrostatic pressure forces plasma water into the interstitial space. After passage of the capillaries 95 % of these fluids will return into the intravascular space. This movement of water is driven by the oncotic pressure gradient, while the remaining interstitial water will return to the circulation as lymphatic fluid. In the peripheral tissue the ion concentration between the plasma volume and the interstital volume is identical and, therefore, it is not an important determinant for fluid exchange. In contrast to the peripheral capillaries, the cerebral capillaries show endothelial tight junctions, which are exclusively permeable for water and impermeable for ions or molecules. Due to this semipermeable membrane in the cerebral and spinal vessels, the so called blood-brain-barrier, fluid exchange between the plasma and the interstitial compartment of central nervous tissue is driven by the osmotic pressure or the plasma-osmolarity (2).

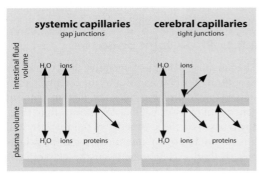

Figure 4.8: Electrolyte transfer along the endothelial barrier.

Osmosis describes the distribution of water depending on the concentration of solved particles on both sides of a membrane, which is impermeable for these particles. With a high concentration of solved particles on one side of the membrane and a low concentration on the other side water will diffuse from the compartment with the low concentration to the compartment with the high concentration until equilibrium. This transfer of water is driven by the osmotic pressure of the particles. Plasma-osmolarity describes the relationship

between the dissolved, osmotically active particles and water. The physiological range of plasma-osmolarity is 280-300 mosmol/l. The sodium ion concentration in the extracellular compartment determinates 90 % of plasma-osmolarity. Therefore, with an intact blood-brain-barrier, the interstitial water volume and the fluid transfer in neuronal tissue is mainly regulated by plasma osmolarity. A decrease in plasma osmolarity (e.g. infusion of free water, hyponatremia) causes filtration of water along the osmotic pressure gradient into the interstitial compartment with consecutive edema formation. In contrast, mild hypernatremia (e.g. following infusion of hypertonic saline) mobilizes interstitial water to move into the vascular space. The infusion of colloid solutions plays only a minor role in the fluid transfer along the blood-brain-barrier (figure 4.8).

4.6.2. Clinically relevant consequences for fluid management in neurosurgical patients

Fluid management in patients with neurosurgical diseases includes a rapid normalization of hypovolemia and the maintenance of a physiological plasma volume (normal heart rate, normal arterial blood pressure, central venous pressure between 8-12 mmHg, jugular bulb saturation higher than 70 %, and a spontaneous urinary output of > 70 mL/h). These conditions are necessary to maintain an adequate cerebral perfusion pressure. The dogma to run neurosurgical patients dry is definitively obsolete, because of the risk of arterial hypotension in these patients (1). At the same time fluid management has to maintain a physiological plasma osmolarity and osmotic pressure to avoid the development of cerebral or spinal edema with consecutive increases in intracranial or intravertebral pressure. These guidelines apply in all patients with intact blood-brain-barrier. After disruption of the blood-brain-barrier by trauma, neoplasm, or infection the characteristics of fluid transfer are unpredictable.

4.6.3. Isotonic solutions: isotonic saline, Ringer´s solution, colloid solutions

In general, any solution is suitable as long as it is iso-osmotic and will stay iso-osmotic after infusion. These criteria are met by isotonic saline (0.9 % NaCl), balanced salt solutions (Ringer's solution), and colloid solutions. Lactated Ringer's solution is almost isotonic. However, in the presence of normal liver function lactate gets metabolized. This will transfer lactated Ringer's solution into a hypo-osmotic solution and generates 8-10 % of free water which will be filtrated along the osmotic gradient into the interstitial space. The amount of water accumulation depends on the amount of infused lactated Ringer's solution. Consequently, in patients with elevated intracranial pressure the upper limit of Ringer's lactate solution per day should not exceed 1000 mL.

4.6.4. Dextrose solution

Dextrose solutions act as free water, because dextrose is metabolized very rapidly. Free water reduces plasma osmolarity, induces fluid transfer from the vascular compartment towards the interstitial space, and causes interstitial and intracellular edema formation. Therefore, dextrose solutions should be used in neurosurgical patients only for treatment of hypoglycemia. Additionally, experimental and clinical studies have shown that hyperglycemia before, during, and after cerebral ischemia or head-trauma worsens neurological outcome due to anaerobic glycolysis (3,4). High plasma-glucose concentrations directly correlate with the degree of anaerobic glycolysis, increasing the cellular and interstitial lactate-concentration with a consecutive decrease of tissue pH. This lactic-acid accumulation increases the permeability of endothelial, glial, and neuronal membranes with water moving into the interstitial and intracellular compartment. This further adds to the impairment of microcirculation. Normoglycemia seems to prevent lactic acidosis and increased membrane permeability and, thereby, protects neuronal tissue during and after hypoxic or ischemic challenges. Plasma glucose concentration should be monitored frequently in neurosurgical patients and maintained between 100-150 mg/dL.

4.6.5. Hypertonic solutions

Hypertonic solutions decrease cerebral and spinal cord water content and improve rheological characteristics. This effect of mannitol leads to a decrease in intracranial pressure, increase in cerebral perfusion pressure and cerebral blood flow (5,6). Therefore, mannitol is the osmotic agent of first choice for reduction of an elevated intracranial

pressure (7). High-dose mannitol appears to be preferable compared to conventional-dose mannitol for the preoperative management of patients with acute subdural hematomas (8,9). Mannitol increases plasma osmolarity and thereby mobilizes interstitial fluid along the osmotic gradient from the intracellular and the interstitial to the intravascular compartment. This counteracts tissue edema formation. The consecutive expansion of the plasma volume decreases hematocrit and viscosity of the blood, which ameliorates perfusion and oxygen delivery in the ischemic regions. The lower blood viscosity reduces the cerebral blood volume by better drainage of the cerebrovenous blood and by autoregulatory vasoconstriction. Additionally, hypertonic solutions mobilize fluid from edematous endothelial cells. This effect promotes the dilation of shock-narrowed capillaries and the restoration of nutritional blood flow. Mannitol may also act as a free radical scavenger. The osmotic effect of mannitol starts 2-30 minutes after infusion. Mannitol should not be used as part of a rigid regimen, preventatively, or continuously by an infusion. In patients with elevated intracranial pressure mannitol should be given as a short infusion (0.25-1.00 g/kg), without exceeding the maximal concentration per day (4.0 g/kg/d) or a plasma osmolarity of more than 320 mOsmol (risk of inducing tubular necrosis). Therefore plasma osmolarity has to be monitored during mannitol therapy. In patients with a defective blood-brain-barrier or with mannitol therapy for more than four days a rebound increase in intracranial pressure is discussed.

Another concept for treatment of high intracranial pressure represents the infusion of hypertonic saline (e.g. 7.5 %). This substance is suitable for small volume resuscitation in patients with multiple injuries and induces an increase in cerebral perfusion pressure and a decrease in intracranial pressure in patients with head trauma (10). Hypertonic saline and mannitol seem to equally reduce intracranial pressure and cerebrospinal fluid pressure (5,11). In patients with posttraumatic intracranial hypertension 2 mL/kg saline 7.5 % decreases intracranial pressure more effectively and for an extended interval than 2 mL/kg mannitol 20 % (12). The combination of hypertonic saline with colloids prolongs the preservation of the gained intravascular volume and has additive beneficial circulatory effects. The administration of hypertonic saline hydroxyethyl starch solution in euvolemic patients reduces elevated intracranial pressure more effectively but does not increase cerebral perfusion pressure as much as mannitol (13). Therefore, hypertonic saline with or without colloids is a valid option in the treatment of intracranial hypertension. However, hypertonic saline should be used carefully because the duration of the treatment, the long-term outcome and the problems of a possible rebound increase of intracranial pressure have not yet been investigated.

4.6.6. Hemodilution (hydroxyethyl starch, dextran, diaspirin cross-linked hemoglobin)

Hypervolemic hemodilution reduces plasma viscosity and might, thereby, improve cerebral blood flow, reduce vascular resistance, and optimize perfusion of ischemic territories. Despite these considerations, patients with focal cerebral ischemia treated with hypervolemic hemodilution (with hydroxyethyl starch or dextran) suffered more hemorrhagic infarcts with a higher lethality compared to non-treated patients (14). Consequently, hypervolemic hemodilution with colloids is contraindicated in patients with pathological cerebral computer tomography scans and acute subarachnoid hemorrhage. Hypervolemic hemodilution in combination with hypertension (triple-H therapy) may reduce the occurrence of vasospasm and death after subarachnoid hemorrhage. However, a systematic review of clinical studies shows that symptomatic vasospasm is less frequent with triple-H therapy after subarachnoid hemorrhage, while the risk of death is higher in these patients (15). Therefore, triple-H therapy for prevention of vasospasm has to be critically discussed.

Hemodilution using a solution with oxygen transporting capacity seems to be superior to colloid solutions. In an experimental study the infusion of diaspirin cross-linked hemoglobin reduced intracranial pressure and infarct size after cerebral ischemia or traumatic brain injury (16,17). In contrast, after severe hemorrhagic shock in pigs with traumatic brain injury diaspirin cross-linked hemoglobin was even less effective than saline resuscitation(18). In patients with severe traumatic hemorrhage shock diaspirin cross-linked hemo-

globin did not reduce morbidity or mortality, in one study mortality was even higher with diaspirin cross-linked hemoglobin (19,20). Therefore, diaspirin cross-linked hemoglobin is not used for blood substitution or hemodilution in patients.

4.6.7. Summary

Increased intracranial pressure and arterial hypotension are the main reasons for increased morbidity and mortality in neurosurgical patients. Consequently, the target of perioperative volume substitution must be a stable normovolemic status. Normovolemia can be achieved by infusion of cristalloid or colloid solutions, which can be isoosmolar or hyperosmolar. Hypotonic solutions and those that will be transferred into hypoosmolar fluids after infusion are contraindicated for volume substitution in neurosurgical patients. Dextrose solutions are exclusively indicated in patients with hypoglycemia. The triple-H therapy (hemodilution, hypertension, and hypervolemia) is only indicated, if at all, in patients with symptomatic vasospasm after subarachnoid hemorrhage.

4.6.8. References

1. Chesnut RM, Marshall LF, Klauber MR, Blunt BA, Baldwin N, Eisenberg HM, Jane JA, Marmarou A, Foulkes MA: The role of secondary brain injury in determining outcome from severe head injury. J Trauma 1993; 34: 216-222

2. Drummond JC, Patel P, Cole DJ, Kelly PJ: The effect of the reduction of colloid oncotic pressure, with and without reduction of osmolality, on post-traumatic cerebral edema. Anesthesiology 1998; 88: 993-1002

3. Woo J, Lam C, Kay R, Wong A, Teoh R, Nicholls M: The influence of hyperglycemia and diabetes mellitus on immediate and 3-month morbidity and mortality after acute stroke. Arch Neurol 1990; 47: 1174-1177

4. De Courten-Myers GM, Kleinholz M, Wagner RE: Normoglycemia (not hypoglycemia) optimizes outcome from middle cerebral artery occlusion. J Cereb Blood Flow Metab 1994; 14: 227-236

5. Freshman SP, Battistella FD, Matteucci M, Wisner DH: Hypertonic saline (7,5 %) versus mannitol: a comparison for treatment of acute head injuries. J Trauma 1993; 35: 344-348

6. Schwartz ML, Tator CH, Rowed DW: A prospective randomized comparison of pentobarbial and mannitol. Can J Neurol Sci 1984; 11: 434-440

7. Smith HP, Kelly DL, McWorther JM, Armstrong D, Johnson R, Transou C, Howard G: Comparison of mannitol regimens in patients with severe head injury undergoing intracranial monitoring. J Neurosurg 1986; 65: 820-824

8. Roberts I, Schierhout G, Wakai A: Mannitol for acute traumatic brain injury (Cochrane review). The Cochrane Library 2003; 3

9. Cruz J, Minoja G, Okuchi K: Improving clinical outcome from acute subdural hematomas with the emergency preoperative administration of high doses of mannitol: a randomized trial. Neurosurgery 2001; 49: 864-871

10. Munar F, Ferrer AM, DeNadal M, Poca MA, Pedraza S, Sahuquillo J, Garnacho A: Cerebral hemodynamic effects of 7.2 % hypertonic saline in patients with head injury and raised intracranial pressure. J Neurotrauma 2000; 17: 41-51

11. Gemma M, Cozzi S, Tommasino C, Mungo M, Calvi MR, Cipriani A, Garancini MP: 7.5 % hypertonic saline versus 20 % mannitol during selective neurosurgical supratentorial procedures. J Neurosug Anesth 1997; 9: 329-334

12. Vialet R, Albanèse J, Thomachot L, Antonini F, Bourgouin A, Alliez B, Martin C: Isovolume hypertonic solutes (sodium chloride or mannitol) in the treatment of refractory posttraumatic intracranial hypertension: 2 ml/kg 7.5 % saline is more effective than 2 ml/kg 20 % mannitol. Crit Care Med 2003; 31: 1683-1687

13. Schwarz S, Schwab S, Bertram M, Aschoff A, Hacke W: Effects of hypertonic saline hydroxyethyl starch solution and mannitol in patients with increased intracranial pressure after stroke. Stroke 1998; 29: 1550-1555

14. Strand T: Evaluation of long-term outcome and safety after hemodilution therapy in acute ischemic stroke. Stroke 1992; 23: 657-662

15. Treggiari MM, Wlader B, Suter PM, Romand JA: Systematic review of the prevention of delayed ischemic neurological deficits with hypertension, hypervolemia, and hemodilution therapy following subarachnoidal hemorrhage. J Neurosug 2003; 98: 978-984

16. Chappell JE,.Shackford SR, McBride WJ: Effect of hemodilution with diaspirin crosslinked hemoglobin on intracranial pressure, cerebral perfusion pressure, and fluid requirements after head injury and shock. J Neurosurg 1997; 86: 131-138

17. Cole DJ, Shell RM, Drummond JC, Reynolds L: Focal cerebral ischemia in rats: effect of hyervolemic hemodilution with diaspirin crosslinked hemoglobin versus albumine on brain injury and edema. Anesthesiology 1993; 78: 335-342

18. Gibson JK, Maxwell RA, Schweitzer JB, Fabian TC, Proctor KG: Resuscitation from severe hemorrhagic shock after traumatic brain injury using saline, shed blood, or a blood substitute. Shock 2002; 17: 234-244

19. Sloan EP, Koenigsberg M, Gens D, Cipolle M, Runge J, Mallory MN, Rodman G: Diaspirin cross-linked hemoglobin (DCLHb) in the treatment of severe traumatic hemorrhagic shock: a randomized controlled efficacy trial. JAMA 1999; 282: 1857-1864

20. Kerner T, Ahlers O, Veit S, Riou B, Saunders M, Pison U: DCL-Hb for tauma patients with severe hemorrhagic shock: the European "on-scene" multicenter study. Intensive Care Med 2003; 29: 378-385

4.7. Volume replacement in cardiac surgery

4.7.1. Introduction

A thorough understanding of what fluids do to the body and what the body reciprocally does to these fluids is indispensable in the cardiac surgical environment. The principle of cardiac anaesthesia is to achieve stable hemodynamics and adequate oxygen deliveries in all circumstances by mastering and integrating all combined effects of fluid therapy, anaesthetic and cardiovascular medication. Patients may present with a wide range of pathophysiological events such as (mild) volume deficits or just the opposite: an overloaded circulation with or without cardiogenic shock, congestive heart failure or pulmonary edema. Disease and medications significantly alter the body-water balance - for example, hypertension, coronary artery disease with normal ventricular function, use of diuretics, and heavy smoking are all associated with reductions in blood volume (11). By contrast, congestive heart failure, renal failure, and hypoproteinemia increase volumes. Obtaining optimal ventricular preloads and preload-reserves require manipulation of different body fluid compartments searching for the "best-fit" between a patient's individual cardiac condition and volume status. The latter may vary consistently depending on preload variations by individual heart-lung and thoracoabdominal interactions under anaesthesia and controlled mechanical ventilation. Besides maintaining optimal levels of stroke volume and organ blood flow, anesthesia-induced disequilibria also have to be corrected. Using peroperative transesophageal echocardiography (TEE) modified preload dependency caused by myocardial hypertrophy and, enlarged or dilated hearts can be appreciated.

A titrated treatment of all body fluid spaces (including third spaces losses) prevents or corrects metabolic disturbances and cellular dysfunction (11). Since there is no uniform approach, clinicians have to consider the pathophysiological conditions and the biochemical mechanisms activated by surgery itself and cardiopulmonary bypass (CPB).

4.7.2. Basic Applied Physiology

4.7.2.1. Cardiac Performance and the Macrocirculation

Frank Starling enunciated in the early 20th century that the energy of ventricular muscle contraction is a function of the length of the muscle fiber. The heart automatically controls its output by the degree of filling: increasing the end-diastolic ventricular volume makes systolic contractions more vigorous to eject greater stroke volumes. The law of Laplace limits volume loading if ventricular dilatation occurs and the heart radius increases. Then, the force needed per myocardial fiber increases (i.e. increased oxygen demand and wall tension) to produce the same pressure necessary to expel a given stroke volume.

According to Arthur Guyton (see Figure 4.9), Mean Circulatory Filling Pressure (P_{MCF}) is the driving energy source of venous return. It is defined as the intravascular pressure equally present everywhere in the circulation under cardiac arrest. The cardiac function controls the right atrial pressure (RAP) and the venous return determines cardiac output. By lowering the outflow pressure (i.e. RAP) the venous return increases. When the RAP drops below the surrounding pleural pressure or atmospheric pressure (i.e. open-thorax) the great veins collapse and venous return is further determined by the factors of the so-called circuit function (12). Besides the P_{MCF} the circuit function includes the following indices:

- the pressure-volume relationship of the venous circulation representing the capacitance with its unstressed and stressed volumes. The stressed volume is the extra fluid, which forces the vessel to stretch its walls above their normal resting shape
- compliance is the inverse of the slope of the pressure-volume relationship and represents changes in volume for a given change in pressure

- the resistance or impedance to the venous return

Since the venous wall tension pressurises the vessels to drive the fluid out, only the stressed volume is important for the returning blood flow. Unstressed volume has to be considered a reservoir, which can be recruited as a homeostatic reserve (12).

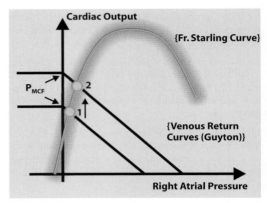

Figure 4.9: Graphical analyse according to Guyton: cardiac output is controlled by the right atrial pressures as the independent variable (x-axis) regulated by the heart and venous return as the dependent variable (y-axis). Extrapolating at a zero venous return, right atrial pressure equals P_{MCF} at the x-intercept. Infusion of volume expands the stressed volume and increases P_{MCF}. Subsequently the venous return curve intersects the cardiac function curve at higher right atrial pressures resulting in an augmented cardiac output (from point 1 to 2).

Changes in resistance provoked by neurosympathetic activation and medication (vasopressors, nitrates, PDE-inhibitors) influence the stressed volume and venous return.

In theory, the ideal monitoring of the volume status would be measuring the P_{MCF}. Unfortunately, its measurements require circulatory arrest. Central venous pressure (CVP) only reflects the interaction of venous return and cardiac function. On the other side, left atrial pressure does not necessarily represent true "filling pressure" since the distensibility of the left ventricle may change. Stroke volume may, therefore, not always increase with rises in right and left atrial pressures. Their value as indicators of volume status is questionable. Swan-Ganz catheter desired cardiac output and pulmonary capillary wedge pressures assess left ventricular function but do not measure peripheral volume reserves. However, less invasive monitoring techniques are currently available (PiCCO™-Pulsion-Germany). Besides a direct measurement of intrathoracic blood volumes and extravascular lung-water this evolving technology also allows the on-line monitoring of beat-to-beat trends of pulse-contour based cardiac output. It further provides indirect estimates of fluid volumes by measuring (ventilation induced) variation of stroke volume and/or pressure to detect the patient's volume responsiveness in combination with consecutive fluid challenges (13).

Position related preload changes can also be appreciated by simply tilting the legs upwards while measuring its impact on cardiovascular performance indices at end-expiration.

Finally, visualizing ventricular chamber size by TEE helps in estimating circulating blood volumes. Moreover, peri-operative TEE is indispensable to diagnose hypertrophy, valvular or congenital disease, enlargement, dilatation and, cardiac contractility. All these factors have important implications for fluid management.

4.7.2.2. Fluid compartments and the microcirculation

Ernest Starling in 1896 determined the forces that distribute fluid between the intravascular and interstitial compartments. The intracapillary hydrostatic pressure is the driving force for fluid filtration out of the intravascular space. Increasing it expands the interstitial volume at the expense of plasma volume, whereas a decrease promotes reabsorption reducing the interstitial volume. This intracapillary pressure represents the link between the micro- and macrocirculation. The so-called Starling-forces that govern fluid movement across the capillary membrane is described by the equation of Starling-Pappenheimer-Staverman in terms of a balance between plasma and tissue colloid osmotic (oncotic) and hydrostatic pressures:

$$Flux_{out} = K_f[\{P_c - P_i\} - S \times \{\pi_c - \pi_i\}]$$

Where π_c and π_i represent the hydrostatic pressures of the capillary and interstitial space, respectively, and π the colloid osmotic (oncotic) pressures of the same compartments; K_f is the filtration coefficient (rate of fluid filtration per mmHg per

100 g tissue expressing the permeability for water) and, S the reflection coefficient reflecting the permeability (1 to 0) for macromolecules.

The intravascular and interstitial compartments together represent the extracellular milieu vis-à-vis the intracellular space. The fluid and composition of the three body-compartments are not static and correspond to their respective contents of osmotic active solutes, mostly electrolytes. Osmotic concentrations of plasma, interstitial fluid, the transcellular fluids and intracellular fluid vary around 300 mosmol/kg. As 1.0 mosmol/kg exerts an osmotic effect of 17 mmHg, the osmotic pressure of the body fluids averages 300 x 17 = 5.100 mmHg. While the capillary wall solely restricts the passage of macromolecules, a Colloid Osmotic Pressure (COP) of 25-30 mm Hg opposes the hydrostatic filtration of fluid to tissue as illustrated in Figure 4.10.

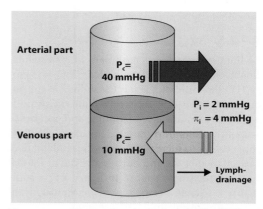

Figure 4.10: The Starling forces include a hydrostatic gradient driving fluids out at the arterial part of the microcirculation, which is counteracted by a colloid osmotic gradient in the opposite direction reabsorbing fluids at the venous part. Overflow is drained by the lymphatic system.

Cell membranes between extra- and extracellular milieu are more restrictive and only permit the free movement of water, which distributes so that its escaping tendency is the same inside in the cell as in the surrounding interstitial fluid.

As shown in Figure 4.11 the intravascular space (IVS) represents the 'acute' space, which is important to be monitored as an end-point for hemodynamic stability. Interstitial and intracellular compartments are only indirectly accessed and manipulated.

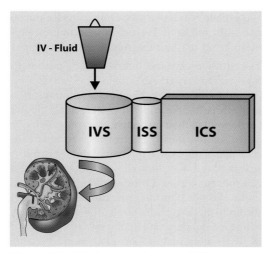

Figure 4.11: The intravascular space (IVS) represents the acute space to which fluids are administered. The kidney regulates the output. The other spaces, the interstitial space (ISS) and intracellular space (ICS) can only indirectly be manipulated.

4.7.2.3. Intravascular Solutions

Sodium is the major determinant of extracellular fluid tonicity and therefore fluids are ISO-, HYPO- or HYPER-tonic with respect to sodium as the reference. HYPO-tonic solutions dilute the osmotic gradient across the cell membrane and water subsequently shifts into the cell. Inversely, HYPER-tonic solutions increase the osmotic gradient over the cell membrane and move water out of the cell to the extracellular spaces. In figure 4.12 a rudimentary scheme shows how to manipulate fluid compartments by fluid replacement.

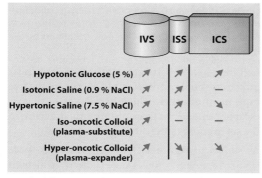

Figure 4.12: Depending on the composition of the fluid infused the different body fluid compartments can be manipulated and either be restored or disturbed.

Thus, by creating an osmotic imbalance between compartments applying suitable solutes intravenously, subsequent water-shifts from one compartment to another can be triggered according to the thermodynamic drive maintaining iso-osmotic conditions over semi-permeable membranes. The infusion of isotonic saline expands the extracellular volume without producing changes in intracellular volume or in intra- or extracellular osmotic concentration. This results from the facts that the osmolality of extracellular fluid is unchanged and that sodium chloride remains mainly extracellular.

Since intravenous solutions also contain electrically charged solutes in an aqueous vehicle, the presence of these charges requires an equal number of cations and anions due to the imperative preservation of electroneutrality. Therefore, unbuffered solutions such as normal saline contain amounts of chloride that exceed the physiological contents, a major cause of (iatrogenic) metabolic acidosis (10). Buffers or their precursors like lactate, acetate, and gluconate are frequently added to reduce this chloride load. Besides their benefits for the acid-base balance, side effects may occur (e.g. lactate induced hyperglycemia).

Based on physiological evidence, body compartments should be restored using solutions imitating more or less the original (ionic and colloidal) composition of each fluid space. Crystalloids are cheap and have no serious adverse effects on patient outcome. However, restoring intravascular hypovolemia only with crystalloid solutions requires larger infused volume (four times that of colloids) to achieve similar haemodynamic effects. Serum COP declines with their use and increases the extravascular water content (interstitial edema) and subsequent organ dysfunction since oxygen transport also depends on the transport through the interstitial space.

Plasma protein derivatives (albumin and the less purified plasma protein fraction) are expensive. Synthetic colloids such as hydroxyethyl starches (HES), gelatins and dextrans represent good alternatives in many cases. Dextran and HES are known to interact with the blood-coagulation system. The respective pharmacological properties, qualities, disadvantage and, also the hazards associated with the different fluids and colloids are reviewed elsewhere.

Data on anaphylactic reactions using colloids are conflicting. Recent studies failed to demonstrate significant differences between colloids in grade III & IV life-threatening reactions (6).

Due to the potential transmission of diseases, homologous blood products are to be reserved to correct anemia or for the treatment of a documented coagulopathy (11).

4.7.2.4. Hemodilution

Isovolemic or hypervolemic dilution of the circulating blood causes a fall in hematocrit and hence a reduction in systemic vascular resistance. The latter results in higher venous return and a rise in cardiac output, if permitted by the cardiac function. There is a proportional increase in cerebral, renal, liver, and intestinal blood flow. The fall in viscosity and resistance is proportionally more important than the decrease in oxygen content. As long as hypovolemia is avoided, supra-maximal values of oxygen transport are obtained at hematocrits around 30 % in basal conditions. This is the cornerstone of all concepts involving isovolemic hemodilution like homologous blood saving programs and rheological therapy.

4.7.2.5. Stewart's biophysical approach to acid-base status

Peter Stewart (14) defined the strong ion gap (SIG), a physical chemical methodology similar to the anion gap (AG). In aqueous solutions, water dissociation is a major source of free hydrogen ions (protons). In this model, bicarbonate and hydrogen ions are considered to be as *dependent variables* and represent the effects (e.g. pH) rather than the causes of acid-base derangements. The three *independent variables* are: pCO_2, weak acids (e.g. proteins and phosphates), and the strong ion difference (SID). SID is the difference between completely dissociated cations (e.g. Na^+) and anions (e.g. Cl^-). H^+ concentration (pH) is determined by the dissociation of water into H^+ and OH^- ions as determined by the physical laws of electro neutrality and conservation of mass. Calculation of the "apparent" SID is as follows:

$$(Na^+ + K^+ + Ca^{++} + Mg^{++}) - (Cl^- + lactate^-)$$

The normal SID value is 40-42 mEq/L. Unmeasured ions might also be present, which results in a Strong Ion Gap (SIG). Colloids in suspension may also be electrically charged like albumin and gelatins, which behave as weak acids in Stewart's analysis. Starches are uncharged and do not contribute to the ionic acid-base equilibrium. The Stewart approach has been validated in the study of cardiopulmonary bypass (CPB)-related acid-base disorders (7,10).

4.7.3. Role of the cardiac anesthesiologist

By combining vasoactive medication with an appropriate fluid replacement strategy patients can be managed towards a stable hemodynamic condition (Figure 4.13).

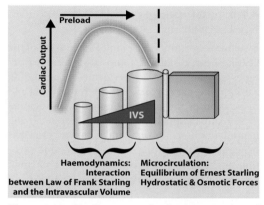

Figure 4.13: 'Starling *versus* Starling': integration of current physiological concepts may help on how to manipulate intravascular fluid space and other fluid compartments in the continuous search for the "best-fit" between a patient's individual cardiac condition and volume status.

Fully-relaxed patients under positive pressure ventilation generally experience a favourable reduction in cardiac afterload. Positional changes of thorax, legs and the body in general also may considerably contribute to better hemodynamics by shifting volumes. Pharmacological (e.g. nitrates and/or phenylephrine) interventions on the venous capacitance, stressed volumes and arterial impedances allow good control when combined with well-chosen and well-timed fluid challenges. Hypertrophic ventricles may benefit from maintaining a good preload and sufficient afterload to prevent collapse and ejection failure. Stunned or hibernating myocardium, dilated or enlarged ventricles are more sensitive to extra preload charges and are commonly favoured by a decreased afterload. Kidney function also can be jeopardized by sustained hypovolemia especially when ACE-inhibitors are used and/or the renal reserve is already impaired. This pre-renal factor for kidney failure should be avoided and monitoring of diuresis is mandatory. The question remains to what level hypovolemia should be corrected (11). After satisfying basal fluid requirements, one should attempt to restore or maintain cardio-dynamic stability to enhance oxygen delivery avoiding anaerobic metabolism and thereby disturbed organ function (11).

4.7.4. Off-pump or on-pump: that's the question

4.7.4.1. Off-pump coronary artery bypass grafting

By temporary immobilization of some areas of the beating heart distal anastomosis on coronary arteries can be performed avoiding cardiopulmonary bypass. However, the lifting and dislocation of the heart combined with regional ischemia may impair cardiac output destabilizing hemodynamics. Empirical and circumstantial evidence shows that tilting down the table and positioning the legs up-right combined with a maximal appropriate intravascular filling and use of vasoactive drugs may produce relative stable cardiodynamic conditions. A good collaboration with an experienced and gentle cardiac surgeon further reduces the need for conversion to cardiopulmonary bypass.

4.7.4.2. Cardiopulmonary Bypass (CPB)

With the initiation of CPB, an extra void is added to the intravascular space by connecting arterial and venous vascular trees to an ex-vivo machinery including plastic tubing, filters, pumps, and an artificial lung. This expansion requires an appropriate solution to fill this extracorporeal circuit. In the early days of CPB, hemodilution using 'clear primes' (using only crystalloids) soon proved to be effective and beneficial in preventing the 'homologous blood syndrome' and postoperative renal problems. Therefore, there is a definite clinical demand for an appropriate substitution to prime (i.e. fill up) the extracorporeal circuit. The sudden mixture of an overwhelming mass of CPB prime with the circulating blood volume definitely modifies its composition. Hemodilution occurs and, if a non-colloid prime is used, there is also a drop in colloid osmotic pressure by the dilution of serum proteins, which results in an expansion of the interstitial space. Although quantitative measurement of how far a solution interferes with the pathophysiological mechanisms is difficult, interplay between the composition of the priming and the CPB-related acid-base disorders has been demonstrated (7). Jansen et al found improved postoperative courses and a reduction in hospital stay using artificial colloids, underlining the importance of maintaining a sufficient colloid osmotic pressure (9). Natural colloids such as human albumin are extremely expensive and there is little evidence to support the routine use of albumin (1). The Systemic Inflammatory Response Syndrome (SIRS) and activation of complement is a consistent phenomenon, that can be reduced by manipulation of the prime (2). Natural colloids are also thought to scavenge oxygen-derived free radicals during ischemia and reperfusion, but clear clinical evidence on this is not available. Evidence on priming fluids in their role as a re-perfusate after de-clamping the aorta favours adding colloids (4). Cardiac performance may also differ depending on what plasma substitute is used during ischaemia and reperfusion (8).

Blood-loss is considered one of the most common and clinically relevant outcomes after cardiac surgery, resulting from either incomplete surgical hemostasis or a CPB-related transient coagulation dysfunction. The recent meta-analysis by Wilkes (5), the retrospective study by Canver (3) and, the earlier review by Cope (5) all demonstrated significantly increased risks of postoperative bleeding when "old" starches are used as plasma-substitutes perioperatively or as pump-primes during cardiac surgery. Whether this is also the case if using these substances when the CPB-related detrimental effects on coagulation are avoided with off-pump cardiac surgery remains to be elucidated. The new generation starches might be more promising in this regard but relevant data are not available yet.

4.7.5. Conclusion

This review offered a limited sample of knowledge on the use of fluids during cardiac surgery. Clinical artistry and individual experience are often re-quired to reach the best outcome. However, more prospective research will be necessary to find out the best mixtures of crystalloids, colloids, and blood-substitutes.

4.7.6. References

1. Boldt J. The good, the bad, and the ugly: should we completely banish human albumin from our intensive care units? Anesth Analg 2000;91:887-95.

2. Bonser RS, Dave JR, Davies ET, et al. Reduction of complement activation during bypass by prime manipulation. Ann Thorac Surg 1990;49:279-83.

3. Canver CC, Nichols RD. Use of intraoperative heta-starch priming during coronary bypass. Chest 2000;118:1616-20.

4. Christlieb IY, Clark RE. Adequacy of the perfusate: Its influence on successful myocardial protection. J Thorac Cardiovasc Surg 1982;84:689-695.

5. Cope JT, Banks D, Mauney MC, et al. Intraoperative hetastarch infusion impairs hemostasis after cardiac operations. Ann Thorac Surg 1997;63:78-83.

6. Himpe D. Allergic reactions to artificial colloids used as plasma substitutes. Ann Fr Anesth Reanim 1995;14:142-3.

7. Himpe D, Neels H, De Hert S, Van Cauwelaert. Adding lactate to the prime solution during hypothermic cardiopulmonary bypass: a quantitative acid-base analysis. Br J Anaesth 2003;90:440-5

8. Himpe DG, De Hert SG, Vermeyen KM, Adriaensen HF. Oxygen transport and myocardial function after the administration of albumin 5 %, hydroxyethylstarch 6 % and succinylated gelatine 4 % to rabbits. Eur J Anaesthesiol 2002;19:860-7.

9. Jansen PG, te Velthuis H, Wildevuur WR, et al. Cardiopulmonary bypass with modified fluid gelatin and heparin-coated circuits. Br J Anaesth 1996;76:13-9.

10. Liskaser FJ, Bellomo R, Hayhoe M, et al. Role of pump prime in the etiology and pathogenesis of cardio-pulmonary bypass-associated acidosis. Anesthesiology 2000;93:1170-3.

11. London MJ. Plasma Volume Expansion in Cardio-vascular Surgery: Practical realities, Theoretical concerns. J Cardiothorac Anesth 1988;2(Suppl1):39-49.

12. Magder S, Scharf S. Venous Return. Lung Biology in Health and Disease 2001;157:93-112.

13. Perel A, Pizov R, Cotev S. Systolic blood pressure variation is a sensitive indicator of hypovolemia in ventilated dogs subjected to graded hemorrhage. Anesthesiology. 1987 Oct;67:498-502.

14. Stewart PA. Modern quantitative acid-base chemistry. Can J Physiol Pharmacol 1983; 61:1444-61

15. Wilkes MM, Navickis RJ, Sibbald WJ., Albumin versus hydroxyethyl starch in cardiopulmonary bypass surgery: a meta-analysis of postoperative bleeding. Ann. Thorac. Surg., 72, 527-34, 2001.

Index

Index